THE SAFETY AND QUALITY OF ABORTION CARE IN THE UNITED STATES

Committee on Reproductive Health Services:
Assessing the Safety and Quality of Abortion Care in the U.S.

Board on Population Health and Public Health Practice

Board on Health Care Services

Health and Medicine Division

A Consensus Study Report of

The National Academies of
SCIENCES · ENGINEERING · MEDICINE

THE NATIONAL ACADEMIES PRESS
Washington, DC
www.nap.edu

THE NATIONAL ACADEMIES PRESS   500 Fifth Street, NW   Washington, DC 20001

This activity was supported by contracts between the National Academy of Sciences and The David and Lucile Packard Foundation, The Grove Foundation, The JPB Foundation, The Susan Thompson Buffett Foundation, Tara Health Foundation, and William and Flora Hewlett Foundation. Any opinions, findings, conclusions, or recommendations expressed in this publication do not necessarily reflect the views of any organization or agency that provided support for the project.

International Standard Book Number-13:   978-0-309-46818-3
International Standard Book Number-10:   0-309-46818-3
Digital Object Identifier: https://doi.org/10.17226/24950
Library of Congress Control Number: 2018939630

Additional copies of this publication are available for sale from the National Academies Press, 500 Fifth Street, NW, Keck 360, Washington, DC 20001; (800) 624-6242 or (202) 334-3313; http://www.nap.edu.

Suggested citation: National Academies of Sciences, Engineering, and Medicine. 2018. *The safety and quality of abortion care in the United States.* Washington, DC: The National Academies Press. doi: https://doi.org/10.17226/24950.

The National Academies of
SCIENCES · ENGINEERING · MEDICINE

The **National Academy of Sciences** was established in 1863 by an Act of Congress, signed by President Lincoln, as a private, nongovernmental institution to advise the nation on issues related to science and technology. Members are elected by their peers for outstanding contributions to research. Dr. Marcia McNutt is president.

The **National Academy of Engineering** was established in 1964 under the charter of the National Academy of Sciences to bring the practices of engineering to advising the nation. Members are elected by their peers for extraordinary contributions to engineering. Dr. C. D. Mote, Jr., is president.

The **National Academy of Medicine** (formerly the Institute of Medicine) was established in 1970 under the charter of the National Academy of Sciences to advise the nation on medical and health issues. Members are elected by their peers for distinguished contributions to medicine and health. Dr. Victor J. Dzau is president.

The three Academies work together as the **National Academies of Sciences, Engineering, and Medicine** to provide independent, objective analysis and advice to the nation and conduct other activities to solve complex problems and inform public policy decisions. The National Academies also encourage education and research, recognize outstanding contributions to knowledge, and increase public understanding in matters of science, engineering, and medicine.

Learn more about the National Academies of Sciences, Engineering, and Medicine at **www.nationalacademies.org**.

The National Academies of
SCIENCES · ENGINEERING · MEDICINE

Consensus Study Reports published by the National Academies of Sciences, Engineering, and Medicine document the evidence-based consensus on the study's statement of task by an authoring committee of experts. Reports typically include findings, conclusions, and recommendations based on information gathered by the committee and the committee's deliberations. Each report has been subjected to a rigorous and independent peer-review process and it represents the position of the National Academies on the statement of task.

Proceedings published by the National Academies of Sciences, Engineering, and Medicine chronicle the presentations and discussions at a workshop, symposium, or other event convened by the National Academies. The statements and opinions contained in proceedings are those of the participants and are not endorsed by other participants, the planning committee, or the National Academies.

For information about other products and activities of the National Academies, please visit www.nationalacademies.org/about/whatwedo.

COMMITTEE ON REPRODUCTIVE HEALTH SERVICES: ASSESSING THE SAFETY AND QUALITY OF ABORTION CARE IN THE U.S.

B. NED CALONGE (*Co-Chair*), University of Colorado
HELENE D. GAYLE (*Co-Chair*), Chicago Community Trust
WENDY R. BREWSTER, University of North Carolina at Chapel Hill School of Medicine
LEE A. FLEISHER, University of Pennsylvania Perelman School of Medicine
CAROL J. ROWLAND HOGUE, Emory University Rollins School of Public Health
JODY RAE LORI, University of Michigan School of Nursing
JEANNE MIRANDA, University of California, Los Angeles
RUTH MURPHEY PARKER, Emory University School of Medicine
DEBORAH E. POWELL, University of Minnesota Medical School
EVA K. PRESSMAN, University of Rochester Medical Center
ALINA SALGANICOFF, Kaiser Family Foundation
PAUL G. SHEKELLE, The RAND Corporation
SUSAN M. WOLF, University of Minnesota

Study Staff

JILL EDEN, Study Director
KATYE MAGEE, Research Associate
MATTHEW MASIELLO, Research Assistant
ANNA MARTIN, Senior Program Assistant
ROSE MARIE MARTINEZ, Senior Director, Board on Population Health and Public Health Practice
SHARYL NASS, Director, Board on Health Care Services
HOPE HARE, Administrative Assistant
PATRICK BURKE, Senior Financial Officer
MISRAK DABI, Financial Associate (*from June 2017*)

Reviewers

This Consensus Study Report was reviewed in draft form by individuals chosen for their diverse perspectives and technical expertise. The purpose of this independent review is to provide candid and critical comments that will assist the National Academies of Sciences, Engineering, and Medicine in making each published report as sound as possible and to ensure that it meets the institutional standards for quality, objectivity, evidence, and responsiveness to the study charge. The review comments and draft manuscript remain confidential to protect the integrity of the deliberative process.

We thank the following individuals for their review of this report:

REBECCA H. ALLEN, Brown University
DONALD M. BERWICK, Institute for Healthcare Improvement
CLAIRE BRINDIS, University of California, San Francisco
PONJOLA CONEY, Virginia Commonwealth University
VANESSA K. DALTON, University of Michigan
C. NEILL EPPERSON, University of Pennsylvania Perelman School of Medicine
DANIEL GROSSMAN, University of California, San Francisco
AMY LEVI, University of New Mexico College of Nursing
HEIDI D. NELSON, Oregon Health & Science University
WILLIE J. PARKER, Physicians for Reproductive Health
ROBERT L. PHILLIPS, JR., American Board of Family Medicine
SARA ROSENBAUM, The George Washington University Milken Institute School of Public Health

MICHAEL W. VARNER, University of Utah School of Medicine
GAIL R. WILENSKY, Project HOPE
SUSAN F. WOOD, The George Washington University

Although the reviewers listed above provided many constructive comments and suggestions, they were not asked to endorse the conclusions or recommendations of this report, nor did they see the final draft before its release. The review of this report was overseen by **ALFRED O. BERG,** University of Washington, and **ENRIQUETA C. BOND,** Burroughs Wellcome Fund. They were responsible for making certain that an independent examination of this report was carried out in accordance with the standards of the National Academies and that all review comments were carefully considered. Responsibility for the final content rests entirely with the authoring committee and the National Academies.

Acknowledgments

The committee and staff are indebted to a number of individuals and organizations for their contributions to this report. We extend special thanks to all the individuals who were essential sources of information, generously giving their time and knowledge to further the committee's efforts. Thank you to Elizabeth Brown, Sidney Callahan, Olivia Cappello, Nancy Chescheir, Mitch Creinin, Carrie Cwiak, Ann Davis, Diana Greene Foster, Marji Gold, Alisa Goldberg, Kristy Goodman, Jane Henney, Susan Higginbotham, Elizabeth Janiak, Tara Jatlaoui, Rachel Jones, Uta Landy, Amy Levi, Steve Lichtenberg, Abigail Long, Ana McKee, Michael Raggio, Matthew Reeves, Debra Stulberg, Diana Taylor, Stephanie Teal, Ushma Upadhyay, Carl Weiner, Kari White, Beverly Winikoff, and Susan Wood.

Thank you as well to the following individuals, who provided testimony to the committee:

BONNIE SCOTT JONES, Senior Policy Advisor, Advancing New Standards in Reproductive Health (ANSIRH), University of California, San Francisco;

SARAH ROBERTS, Associate Professor, ANSIRH, Department of Obstetrics, Gynecology, and Reproductive Sciences, University of California, San Francisco; and

JULIET ROGERS, Assistant Professor, Health Management and Policy, University of Michigan.

Funding for this study was provided by The David and Lucile Packard Foundation, The Grove Foundation, The JPB Foundation, The Susan Thompson Buffett Foundation, Tara Health Foundation, and William and Flora Hewlett Foundation. The committee appreciates the opportunity and support extended by the sponsors for the development of this report.

Many within the Health and Medicine Division (HMD) of the National Academies of Sciences, Engineering, and Medicine were helpful to the study staff. The committee would like to thank Rebecca Morgan and the National Academies Research Center staff for their assistance in the committee's research efforts. We would also like to thank Patrick Burke and Misrak Dabi (HMD Offices of Finance and Administration); Chelsea Frakes, Lauren Shern, and Taryn Young (HMD Executive Office); and Greta Gorman, Nicole Joy, and Bettina Ritter (HMD Office of Communications).

Contents

Boxes, Figures, and Tables

Summary[1]

When the Institute of Medicine (IOM)[2] issued its 1975 report on the public health impact of legalized abortion, the scientific evidence on the safety and health effects of legal abortion services was limited. It had been only 2 years since the landmark *Roe v. Wade* decision had legalized abortion throughout the United States, and nationwide data collection was just under way. Today, the available evidence on abortion's health effects is quite robust. There is a great deal of related scientific research, including well-designed randomized controlled trials, systematic reviews, and epidemiological studies examining the relative safety of abortion methods and the appropriateness of methods for different clinical circumstances. With this growing body of research, medical and surgical abortion methods have been refined or discontinued, and new techniques have been developed.

In 2016, six private foundations came together to ask the Health and Medicine Division of the National Academies of Sciences, Engineering, and Medicine to conduct a comprehensive review of the state of the science on the safety and quality of legal abortion services in the United States. The sponsors—The David and Lucile Packard Foundation, The Grove Foundation, The JPB Foundation, The Susan Thompson Buffett Foundation, Tara Health Foundation, and William and Flora Hewlett Foundation—asked

---

[1]This summary does not include references. Relevant citations appear in subsequent chapters.

[2]In March 2016, the division of the National Academies of Sciences, Engineering, and Medicine that focuses on health and medicine, previously known as the Institute of Medicine (IOM), was renamed the Health and Medicine Division.

1

that the review focus on the eight research questions listed in Box S-1. The Committee on Reproductive Health Services: Assessing the Safety and Quality of Abortion Care in the U.S. was appointed in December 2016 to conduct the study and prepare this report.

BOX S-1
Charge to the Committee on Reproductive Health Services:
Assessing the Safety and Quality of Abortion Care in the U.S.

In 1975, the Institute of Medicine (IOM) issued the report *Legalized Abortion and the Public Health: Report of a Study*. The report contained a comprehensive analysis of the then available scientific evidence on the impact of abortion on the health of the public. Since 1975, there have been substantial changes in the U.S. health care delivery system and in medical science. In addition, practices for abortion care have changed, including the introduction of new techniques and technologies. An updated systematic and independent analysis of today's available evidence has not been conducted. An ad hoc consensus committee of the Health and Medicine Division, which as of March 2016 continues the consensus studies and convening activities previously carried out by the IOM, will produce a comprehensive report on the current state of the science related to the provision of safe, high-quality abortion services in the United States.

The committee will consider the following questions and offer findings and recommendations:

1. What types of legal abortion services are available in the United States? What is the evidence regarding which services are appropriate under different clinical circumstances (e.g., based on patient medical conditions such as previous cesarean section, obesity, gestational age)?
2. What is the evidence on the physical and mental health risks of these different abortion interventions?
3. What is the evidence on the safety and quality of medical and surgical abortion care?
4. What is the evidence on the minimum characteristics of clinical facilities necessary to effectively and safely provide the different types of abortion interventions?
5. What is the evidence on what clinical skills are necessary for health care providers to safely perform the various components of abortion care, including pregnancy determination, counseling, gestational age assessment, medication dispensing, procedure performance, patient monitoring, and follow-up assessment and care?
6. What safeguards are necessary to manage medical emergencies arising from abortion interventions?
7. What is the evidence on the safe provision of pain management for abortion care?
8. What are the research gaps associated with the provision of safe, high-quality care from pre- to postabortion?

CONTEXT FOR THIS REPORT

What Is Quality Abortion Care?

The committee agreed that two fundamental principles would guide its work: first, that women should expect that the abortion care they receive meets well-established clinical standards for objectivity, transparency, and scientific rigor; and second, that the quality of abortion care should be assessed using the six dimensions of health care quality first described in the 2001 IOM report *Crossing the Quality Chasm: A New Health System for the 21st Century* (see Box S-2). These dimensions—safety, effectiveness, patient-centeredness, timeliness, efficiency, and equity—have guided public and private efforts to improve U.S. health care delivery at the local, state, and national levels for more than 15 years. Donabedian's structure-process-outcome framework was also foundational for this report. Figure S-1 illustrates the committee's adaptation of these concepts for assessing abortion care.

BOX S-2
The Six Dimensions of Health Care Quality

Crossing the Quality Chasm: A New Health System for the 21st Century

1. Safety—avoiding injuries to patients from the care that is intended to help them.

2. Effectiveness—providing services based on scientific knowledge to all who could benefit and refraining from providing services to those not likely to benefit (avoiding underuse and overuse, respectively).

3. Patient-centeredness—providing care that is respectful of and responsive to individual patient preferences, needs, and values and ensuring that patient values guide all clinical decisions.

4. Timeliness—reducing waits and sometimes harmful delays for both those who receive and those who give care.

5. Efficiency—avoiding waste, including waste of equipment, supplies, ideas, and energy.

6. Equity—providing care that does not vary in quality because of personal characteristics such as gender, ethnicity, geographic location, and socioeconomic status.

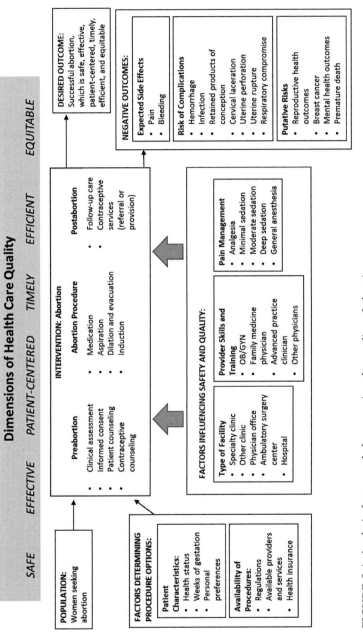

FIGURE S-1 Analytic framework for assessing the quality of abortion care.
NOTE: OB/GYN = obstetrician/gynecologist.

Trends

In the immediate years after national legalization, legal abortions increased steadily until peaking in the 1980s. Since then, there has been a steady decline in both the annual number and rate of abortions. Between 1980 and 2014, the abortion rate among U.S. women fell by more than half, from 29.3 to 14.6 per 1,000 women. In 2014, the aggregate number of abortions reached a low of 926,190. The reason for these declines is not fully understood, but they have been attributed to the increasing use of contraceptives, especially long-acting methods (e.g., intrauterine devices [IUDs] and implants), historic declines in the rate of unintended pregnancy, and increasing numbers of state regulations that limit the availability of otherwise legal abortion services.

Since national legalization, most abortions in the United States (91.6 percent) have been performed in early pregnancy (i.e., ≤13 weeks). With advances in technology such as highly sensitive pregnancy tests and the availability of medication abortion, abortions are being performed at increasingly earlier gestation. According to the Centers for Disease Control and Prevention, the percentage of early abortions performed at ≤6 weeks' gestation increased by 16 percent from 2004 to 2013. In 2013, 38 percent of early abortions occurred at ≤6 weeks' gestation. The proportion of early-gestation abortions occurring at ≤6 weeks is expected to increase even further as the use of medication abortion becomes more common.

Abortion Methods

Abortion methods have evolved and improved in the decades since national legalization. Four legal abortion methods—medication,[3] aspiration, dilation and evacuation (D&E), and induction—are used in the United States. Today, aspiration is the most common abortion method used in the United States, accounting for almost 68 percent of abortions performed overall in 2013. Its use, however, is likely to decline as the use of medication abortion increases. The percentage of total abortions by the medication method rose from 10.6 to 22.3 percent between 2004 and 2013. In 2014, approximately 45 percent of abortions up to 9 weeks' gestation were medication abortions, up from 36 percent in 2011. Fewer than 9 percent of abortions are performed after 13 weeks' gestation—typically by D&E. In 2013, approximately 2 percent of U.S. abortions at 14 weeks' gestation or later were induction procedures.

---

[3]The terms "medication abortion" and "medical abortion" are used interchangeably in the literature. This report uses "medication abortion" to describe the U.S. Food and Drug Administration (FDA)-approved prescription drug regimen used up to 10 weeks' gestation.

Clinical Settings

In 2014, the vast majority of abortions were performed in nonhospital settings: either an abortion clinic (59 percent) or a clinic offering a variety of medical services (36 percent). Fewer than 5 percent of abortions were provided in hospitals.

The overall number of facilities providing abortions—especially specialty abortion clinics—is declining. The greatest proportional decline is in states that have enacted abortion-specific regulations. In 2014, there were 272 abortion clinics in the United States—17 percent fewer than in 2011— and 39 percent of women of reproductive age resided in a county without an abortion provider. Twenty-five states have five or fewer abortion clinics; five states have only one abortion clinic. An estimated 17 percent of women travel more than 50 miles to obtain an abortion.

Women Who Have Abortions

Most women who have abortions are under age 30 (72 percent), are unmarried (86 percent), and are poor or low income (75 percent). Women who have abortions are also more likely to be women of color[4] (61.0 percent); half of all women who have abortions are black (24.8 percent) or Hispanic (24.5 percent). This distribution is similar to the racial and ethnic distribution of women with household incomes below 200 percent of the federal poverty level (FPL). Poor women and women of color are also more likely than others to experience an unintended pregnancy.

Unique Regulatory Environment

Abortion is among the most regulated medical procedures in the nation. While a comprehensive legal analysis of abortion regulation is beyond the scope of this report, the committee agreed that it should consider how abortion's unique regulatory environment relates to the safety and quality of abortion care. Federal restrictions on the distribution of mifepristone (one of the drugs used in medication abortion) also merit attention given its increasing use and the extensive body of research demonstrating its safety and effectiveness.

State Regulations

States play an essential role in ensuring the safety of health care services, especially through their licensure of clinicians and health care facilities. In

---

[4]Includes all nonwhite races and ethnicities.

every state, clinicians and inpatient facilities (e.g., hospitals, rehabilitation centers) must be licensed by a state board or agency to provide health care services legally. When states regulate specific office-based health care procedures, the requirements are usually triggered by the level of sedation that the facility offers. Abortion services are an exception. A wide variety of state regulations affect abortion care, including the type of clinician permitted to perform an abortion, independently of the relevant scope of practice laws (e.g., qualified advanced practice clinicians [APCs] or physicians without hospital privileges may be barred from performing abortions); health insurance coverage (e.g., Medicaid or private insurance plans may be prohibited from paying for abortions); how the informed consent process is conducted (e.g., providers may be required to inform women that abortion increases their risk of breast cancer or mental illness, despite the absence of valid scientific evidence); the abortion method that is used (e.g., D&Es may be banned); the timing and scheduling of procedures (e.g., women may have to wait 18 to 72 hours after a counseling appointment); and the physical attributes of the clinical setting (e.g., procedure room size, corridor width). In most states, the regulations apply to all abortion methods regardless of weeks' gestation, the use of sedation, or the invasiveness of the procedure.

U.S. Food and Drug Administration's (FDA's) Risk Evaluation and Mitigation Strategy (REMS) Program

The distribution and use of mifepristone has been restricted under the requirements of the FDA's REMS program since 2011. The FDA-approved protocol for medication abortion was updated in 2016 based on extensive clinical research demonstrating the safety of the revised regimen. The revised REMS continues to limit the distribution of Mifeprex (the brand name for mifepristone) to patients in clinics, hospitals, or medical offices under the supervision of a certified prescriber and cannot be sold in retail pharmacies. The committee could not find evidence on how this restriction impacts the safety or quality of abortions.

CONCLUSIONS

This report provides a comprehensive review of the state of the science on the safety and quality of abortion services in the United States. As noted earlier (see Box S-1), the committee was charged with answering eight specific research questions. The committee's conclusions regarding each question appear below. The committee was also asked to offer recommendations regarding the eight questions. However, the committee decided that its conclusions regarding the safety and quality of U.S. abortion care responded comprehensively to the scope of this study. Therefore, the committee does not offer recommendations for specific actions to be taken by policy makers, health care providers, and others.

The Research Questions

1. *What types of legal abortion services are available in the United States? What is the evidence regarding which services are appropriate under different clinical circumstances (e.g., based on patient medical conditions such as previous cesarean section, obesity, gestational age)?*

As noted above, four legal abortion methods—medication, aspiration, D&E, and induction—are used in the United States. Length of gestation—measured as the amount of time since the first day of the last menstrual period—is the primary factor in deciding which abortion procedure is the most appropriate. Both medication and aspiration abortions are used up to 10 weeks' gestation. Aspiration procedures may be used up to 14 to 16 weeks' gestation.

Mifepristone, which, as noted above, is sold under the brand name Mifeprex, is the only medication specifically approved by the FDA for use in medication abortion. As discussed earlier, the drug's distribution has been restricted under the requirements of the FDA REMS program since 2011—it may be dispensed only to patients in clinics, hospitals, or medical offices under the supervision of a certified prescriber. To become a certified prescriber, eligible clinicians must register with the drug's distributor, Danco Laboratories, and meet certain requirements. Retail pharmacies are prohibited from distributing the drug.

When abortion by aspiration is no longer feasible, D&E and induction methods are used. D&E is the superior method; in comparison, inductions are more painful for women, take significantly more time, and are more costly. However, D&Es are not always available to women. The procedure is illegal in Mississippi and West Virginia.[5] Elsewhere, access to the procedure is limited because many obstetrician/gynecologists (OB/GYNs) and other physicians lack the requisite training to perform D&Es. Physicians' access to D&E training is very limited or nonexistent in many areas of the country.

Few women are medically ineligible for abortion. There are, however, specific contraindications to using mifepristone for a medication abortion or induction. The drug should not be used for women with confirmed or suspected ectopic pregnancy or undiagnosed adnexal mass; an IUD in place; chronic adrenal failure; concurrent long-term systemic corticosteroid

---

[5]Both states allow exceptions in cases of life endangerment or severe physical health risk to the woman.

therapy; hemorrhagic disorders or concurrent anticoagulant therapy; allergy to mifepristone, misoprostol, or other prostaglandins; or inherited porphyrias.

Obesity is not a risk factor for women who undergo medication or aspiration abortions (including with the use of moderate intravenous sedation). Research on the association between obesity and complications during a D&E abortion is less certain—particularly for women with Class III obesity (body mass index ≥40) after 14 weeks' gestation.

A history of a prior cesarean delivery is not a risk factor for women undergoing medication or aspiration abortions, but it may be associated with an increased risk of complications during D&E abortions, particularly for women with multiple cesarean deliveries. Because induction abortions are so rare, it is difficult to determine definitively whether a prior cesarean delivery increases the risk of complications. The available research suggests no association.

2. What is the evidence on the physical and mental health risks of these different abortion interventions?

Abortion has been investigated for its potential long-term effects on future childbearing and pregnancy outcomes, risk of breast cancer, mental health disorders, and premature death. The committee found that much of the published literature on these topics does not meet scientific standards for rigorous, unbiased research. Reliable research uses documented records of a prior abortion, analyzes comparable study and control groups, and controls for confounding variables shown to affect the outcome of interest.

Physical health effects   The committee identified high-quality research on numerous outcomes of interest and concludes that having an abortion does not increase a woman's risk of secondary infertility, pregnancy-related hypertensive disorders, abnormal placentation (after a D&E abortion), preterm birth, or breast cancer. Although rare, the risk of very preterm birth (<28 weeks' gestation) in a woman's first birth was found to be associated with having two or more prior aspiration abortions compared with first births among women with no abortion history; the risk appears to be associated with the number of prior abortions. Preterm birth is associated with pregnancy spacing after an abortion: it is more likely if the interval between abortion and conception is less than 6 months (this is also true of pregnancy spacing in general). The committee did not find well-designed research on abortion's association with future ectopic pregnancy, miscarriage or stillbirth, or long-term mortality. Findings on hemorrhage during a subsequent pregnancy are inconclusive.

Mental health effects   The committee identified a wide array of research on whether abortion increases women's risk of depression, anxiety, and/or posttraumatic stress disorder and concludes that having an abortion does not increase a woman's risk of these mental health disorders.

3. *What is the evidence on the safety and quality of medical and surgical abortion care?*

Safety   The clinical evidence clearly shows that legal abortions in the United States—whether by medication, aspiration, D&E, or induction—are safe and effective. Serious complications are rare. But the risk of a serious complication increases with weeks' gestation. As the number of weeks increases, the invasiveness of the required procedure and the need for deeper levels of sedation also increase.

Quality   Health care quality is a multidimensional concept. As noted above, six attributes of health care quality—safety, effectiveness, patient-centeredness, timeliness, efficiency, and equity—were central to the committee's review of the quality of abortion care. Table S-1 details the committee's conclusions regarding each of these quality attributes. Overall, the committee concludes that the quality of abortion care depends to a great extent on where women live. In many parts of the country, state regulations have created barriers to optimizing each dimension of quality care. The quality of care is optimal when the care is based on current evidence and when trained clinicians are available to provide abortion services.

4. *What is the evidence on the minimum characteristics of clinical facilities necessary to effectively and safely provide the different types of abortion interventions?*

Most abortions can be provided safely in office-based settings. No special equipment or emergency arrangements are required for medication abortions. For other abortion methods, the minimum facility characteristics depend on the level of sedation that is used. Aspiration abortions are performed safely in office and clinic settings. If moderate sedation is used, the facility should have emergency resuscitation equipment and an emergency transfer plan, as well as equipment to monitor oxygen saturation, heart rate, and blood pressure. For D&Es that involve deep sedation or general anesthesia, the facility should be similarly equipped and also have equipment to provide general anesthesia and monitor ventilation.

Women with severe systemic disease require special measures if they desire or need deep sedation or general anesthesia. These women require

TABLE S-1 Does Abortion Care in the United States Meet the Six Attributes of Quality Health Care?

Quality Attribute[a]	Definition	Committee's Conclusions
Safety	Avoiding injuries to patients from the care that is intended to help them.	Legal abortions—whether by medication, aspiration, D&E, or induction—are safe. Serious complications are rare and occur far less frequently than during childbirth. Safety is enhanced when the abortion is performed as early in pregnancy as possible.
Effectiveness[b]	Providing services based on scientific knowledge to all who could benefit and refraining from providing services to those not likely to benefit (avoiding underuse and overuse, respectively).	Legal abortions—whether by medication, aspiration, D&E, or induction—are effective. The likelihood that women will receive the type of abortion services that best meet their needs varies considerably depending on where they live. In many parts of the country, abortion-specific regulations on the site and nature of care, provider type, provider training, and public funding diminish this dimension of quality care. The regulations may limit the number of available providers, misinform women of the risks of the procedures they are considering, overrule women's and clinician's medical decision making, or require medically unnecessary services and delays in care. These include policies that • require office-based settings to meet the structural standards of higher-intensity clinical facilities (e.g., ambulatory surgery centers or hospitals) even for the least invasive abortion methods (medication and aspiration); • prohibit the abortion method that is most effective for a particular clinical circumstance (e.g., D&E); • delay care unnecessarily from a clinical standpoint (e.g., mandatory waiting periods); • prohibit qualified clinicians (family medicine physicians, certified nurse-midwives, nurse practitioners, and physician assistants) from performing abortions; • require the informed consent process to include inaccurate information on abortion's long-term physical and mental health effects; • require individual clinicians to have hospital privileges; • bar publicly funded clinics from providing abortion care to low-income women; or • mandate clinically unnecessary services (e.g., preabortion ultrasound, in-person counseling visit).

continued

TABLE S-1 Continued

Quality Attribute[a]	Definition	Committee's Conclusions
Patient-Centeredness	Providing care that is respectful of and responsive to individual patient preferences, needs, and values and ensuring that patient values guide all clinical decisions.	Patients' personal circumstances and individual preferences (including preferred abortion method), needs, and values may be disregarded depending on where they live (as noted above). The high state-to-state variability regarding the specifics of abortion care may be difficult for patients to understand and navigate. Patients' ability to be adequately informed in order to make sound medical decisions is impeded when state regulations require that • women be provided inaccurate or misleading information about abortion's potential harms; and • women's preferences for whether they want individualized counseling not be taken into consideration.
Timeliness	Reducing waits and sometimes harmful delays for both those who receive and those who give care.	The timeliness of an abortion depends on a variety of local factors, such as the availability of care, affordability, distance from the provider, and state requirements for an in-person counseling appointment and waiting periods (18 to 72 hours) between counseling and the abortion. • There is some evidence that the logistical challenges of arranging and getting to a second appointment can result in delaying the abortion procedure beyond the mandatory waiting period. • Delays put the patient at greater risk of an adverse event.
Efficiency	Avoiding waste, including waste of equipment, supplies, ideas, and energy.	An extensive body of clinical research has led to important refinements and improvements in the procedures, techniques, and methods for performing abortions. The extent to which abortion care is delivered efficiently depends, in part, on the alignment of state regulations with current evidence on best practices. Regulations that require medically unnecessary equipment, services, and/or additional patient visits increase cost, and thus decrease efficiency.

TABLE S-1 Continued

Quality Attribute[a]	Definition	Committee's Conclusions
Equity	Providing care that does not vary in quality because of personal characteristics such as gender, ethnicity, geographic location, and socioeconomic status.	State-level abortion regulations are likely to affect women differently based on their geographic location and socioeconomic status. Barriers (lack of insurance coverage, waiting periods, limits on qualified providers, and requirements for multiple appointments) are more burdensome for women who reside far from providers and/or have limited resources. • Women who undergo abortions are disproportionately lower-income compared with other women of similar age: family incomes of 49 percent of them are below the federal poverty level (FPL), and family incomes of 26 percent are 100 to 200 percent of the FPL; 61 percent are women of color. • Seventeen percent of women travel more than 50 miles to obtain an abortion.

[a]These attributes of quality health care were first proposed by the Institute of Medicine's Committee on Quality of Health Care in America in the 2001 report *Crossing the Quality Chasm: A New Health System for the 21st Century.*
[b]Elsewhere in this report, effectiveness refers to the successful completion of the abortion without the need for a follow-up aspiration.

further clinical assessment and should have their abortion in either an accredited ambulatory surgery center or hospital.

5. *What is the evidence on what clinical skills are necessary for health care providers to safely perform the various components of abortion care, including pregnancy determination, counseling, gestational age assessment, medication dispensing, procedure performance, patient monitoring, and follow-up assessment and care?*

Required skills All abortion procedures require competent providers skilled in patient preparation (education, counseling, and informed consent); clinical assessment (confirming intrauterine pregnancy, determining gestation, taking a relevant medical history, and physical examination); pain management; identification and management of expected side effects and serious complications; and contraceptive counseling and provision. To provide medication abortions, the clinician should be skilled in all these areas. To provide aspiration abortions, the clinician should also be skilled in the technical aspects of an aspiration procedure. To provide D&E abortions, the clinician needs the relevant surgical expertise and sufficient caseload to maintain the requisite surgical skills. To provide induction abortions, the clinician requires the skills needed for managing labor and delivery.

Clinicians that have the necessary competencies   Both trained physicians (OB/GYNs, family medicine physicians, and other physicians) and APCs (physician assistants, certified nurse-midwives, and nurse practitioners) can provide medication and aspiration abortions safely and effectively. OB/GYNs, family medicine physicians, and other physicians with appropriate training and experience can provide D&E abortions. Induction abortions can be provided by clinicians (OB/GYNs, family medicine physicians, and certified nurse-midwives) with training in managing labor and delivery.

The extensive body of research documenting the safety of abortion care in the United States reflects the outcomes of abortions provided by thousands of individual clinicians. The use of sedation and anesthesia may require special expertise. If moderate sedation is used, it is essential to have a nurse or other qualified clinical staff—in addition to the person performing the abortion—available to monitor the patient, as is the case for any other medical procedure. Deep sedation and general anesthesia require the expertise of an anesthesiologist or certified registered nurse anesthetist to ensure patient safety.

6.   *What safeguards are necessary to manage medical emergencies arising from abortion interventions?*

The key safeguards—for abortions and all outpatient procedures—are whether the facility has the appropriate equipment, personnel, and emergency transfer plan to address any complications that might occur. No special equipment or emergency arrangements are required for medication abortions; however, clinics should provide a 24-hour clinician-staffed telephone line and have a plan to provide emergency care to patients after hours. If moderate sedation is used during an aspiration abortion, the facility should have emergency resuscitation equipment and an emergency transfer plan, as well as equipment to monitor oxygen saturation, heart rate, and blood pressure. D&Es that involve deep sedation or general anesthesia should be provided in similarly equipped facilities that also have equipment to monitor ventilation.

The committee found no evidence indicating that clinicians that perform abortions require hospital privileges to ensure a safe outcome for the patient. Providers should, however, be able to provide or arrange for patient access or transfer to medical facilities equipped to provide blood transfusions, surgical intervention, and resuscitation, if necessary.

7. What is the evidence on the safe provision of pain management for abortion care?

Nonsteroidal anti-inflammatory drugs (NSAIDs) are recommended to reduce the discomfort of pain and cramping during a medication abortion. Some women still report high levels of pain, and researchers are exploring new ways to provide prophylactic pain management for medication abortion. The pharmaceutical options for pain management during aspiration, D&E, and induction abortions range from local anesthesia, to minimal sedation/anxiolysis, to moderate sedation/analgesia, to deep sedation/analgesia, to general anesthesia. Along this continuum, the physiological effects of sedation have increasing clinical implications and, depending on the depth of sedation, may require special equipment and personnel to ensure the patient's safety. The greatest risk of using sedative agents is respiratory depression. The vast majority of abortion patients are healthy and medically eligible for all levels of sedation in office-based settings. As noted above (see Questions 4 and 6), if sedation is used, the facility should be appropriately equipped and staffed.

8. What are the research gaps associated with the provision of safe, high-quality care from pre- to postabortion?

The committee's overarching task was to assess the safety and quality of abortion care in the United States. The committee decided that its findings and conclusions fully respond to this charge. The committee concludes that legal abortions are safe and effective. Safety and quality are optimized when the abortion is performed as early in pregnancy as possible. Quality requires that care be respectful of individual patient preferences, needs, and values so that patient values guide all clinical decisions.

The committee did not identify gaps in research that raise concerns about these conclusions and does not offer recommendations for specific actions to be taken by policy makers, health care providers, and others.

The following are the committee's observations about questions that merit further investigation.

Limitation of Mifepristone distribution   Mifepristone (Mifeprex) is the only medication approved by the FDA for use in medication abortion. Extensive clinical research has demonstrated its safety and effectiveness using the FDA-recommended regimen. Furthermore, few women have contraindications to medication abortion. Nevertheless, as noted earlier, the FDA REMS restricts the distribution of mifepristone. Research is needed on how the limited distribution of mifepristone under the REMS process impacts dimensions of quality, including timeliness, patient-centeredness, and equity. In addition, little is known about pharmacist and patient perspectives on pharmacy dispensing of mifepristone and the potential for direct-to-patient models through telemedicine.

Pain management There is insufficient evidence to identify the optimal approach to minimizing the pain women experience during an aspiration procedure without sedation. Paracervical blocks are effective in decreasing procedural pain, but the administration of the block itself is painful, and even with the block, women report experiencing moderate to significant pain. More research is needed to learn how best to reduce the pain women experience during abortion procedures.

Research on prophylactic pain management for women undergoing medication abortions is also needed. Although NSAIDs reduce the pain of cramping, women still report high levels of pain.

Availability of providers APCs can provide medication and aspiration abortions safely and effectively, but the committee did not find research assessing whether APCs can also be trained to perform D&Es.

Addressing the needs of women of lower income Women who have abortions are disproportionately poor and at risk for interpersonal and other types of violence. Yet little is known about the extent to which they receive needed social and psychological supports when seeking abortion care or how best to meet those needs. More research is needed to assess the need for support services and to define best clinical practice for providing those services.

1

Introduction

When the Institute of Medicine (IOM)[1] issued its 1975 report on the public health impact of legalized abortion, the scientific evidence on the safety and health effects of legal abortion services was limited (IOM, 1975). It had been only 2 years since the landmark *Roe v. Wade* decision had legalized abortion throughout the United States and nationwide data collection was just under way (Cates et al., 2000; Kahn et al., 1971). Today, the available scientific evidence on abortion's health effects is quite robust.

In 2016, six private foundations came together to ask the Health and Medicine Division of the National Academies of Sciences, Engineering, and Medicine to conduct a comprehensive review of the state of the science on the safety and quality of legal abortion services in the United States. The sponsors—The David and Lucile Packard Foundation, The Grove Foundation, The JPB Foundation, The Susan Thompson Buffett Foundation, Tara Health Foundation, and William and Flora Hewlett Foundation—asked that the review focus on the eight research questions listed in Box 1-1.

The Committee on Reproductive Health Services: Assessing the Safety and Quality of Abortion Care in the U.S. was appointed in December 2016 to conduct the study and prepare this report. The committee included 13 individuals[2] with research or clinical experience in anesthesiology,

---

[1] In March 2016, the IOM, the division of the National Academies of Sciences, Engineering, and Medicine focused on health and medicine, was renamed the Health and Medicine Division.

[2] A 14th committee member participated for just the first 4 months of the study.

BOX 1-1
Charge to the Committee on Reproductive Health Services:
Assessing the Safety and Quality of Abortion Care in the U.S.

In 1975, the Institute of Medicine (IOM) issued the report *Legalized Abortion and the Public Health: Report of a Study.* The report contained a comprehensive analysis of the then available scientific evidence on the impact of abortion on the health of the public. Since 1975, there have been substantial changes in the U.S. health care delivery system and in medical science. In addition, practices for abortion care have changed, including the introduction of new techniques and technologies. An updated systematic and independent analysis of today's available evidence has not been conducted. An ad hoc consensus committee of the Health and Medicine Division, which as of March 2016 continues the consensus studies and convening activities previously carried out by the IOM, will produce a comprehensive report on the current state of the science related to the provision of safe, high-quality abortion services in the United States.

The committee will consider the following questions and offer findings and recommendations:

1. What types of legal abortion services are available in the United States? What is the evidence regarding which services are appropriate under different clinical circumstances (e.g., based on patient medical conditions such as previous cesarean section, obesity, gestational age)?
2. What is the evidence on the physical and mental health risks of these different abortion interventions?
3. What is the evidence on the safety and quality of medical and surgical abortion care?
4. What is the evidence on the minimum characteristics of clinical facilities necessary to effectively and safely provide the different types of abortion interventions?
5. What is the evidence on what clinical skills are necessary for health care providers to safely perform the various components of abortion care, including pregnancy determination, counseling, gestational age assessment, medication dispensing, procedure performance, patient monitoring, and follow-up assessment and care?
6. What safeguards are necessary to manage medical emergencies arising from abortion interventions?
7. What is the evidence on the safe provision of pain management for abortion care?
8. What are the research gaps associated with the provision of safe, high-quality care from pre- to postabortion?

---

obstetrics and gynecology, nursing and midwifery, primary care, epidemiology of reproductive health, mental health, health care disparities, health care delivery and management, health law, health professional education and training, public health, quality assurance and assessment, statistics and research methods, and women's health policy. Brief biographies of committee members are provided in Appendix A.

This chapter describes the context for the study and the scope of the inquiry. It also presents the committee's conceptual framework for conducting its review.

ABORTION CARE TODAY

Since the IOM first reviewed the health implications of national legalized abortion in 1975, there has been a plethora of related scientific research, including well-designed randomized controlled trials (RCTs), systematic reviews, and epidemiological studies examining abortion care. This research has focused on examining the relative safety of abortion methods and the appropriateness of methods for different clinical circumstances (Ashok et al., 2004; Autry et al., 2002; Bartlett et al., 2004; Borgatta, 2011; Borkowski et al., 2015; Bryant et al., 2011; Cates et al., 1982; Chen and Creinin, 2015; Cleland et al., 2013; Frick et al., 2010; Gary and Harrison, 2006; Grimes et al., 2004; Grossman et al., 2008, 2011; Ireland et al., 2015; Kelly et al., 2010; Kulier et al., 2011; Lohr et al., 2008; Low et al., 2012; Mauelshagen et al., 2009; Ngoc et al., 2011; Ohannessian et al., 2016; Peterson et al., 1983; Raymond et al., 2013; Roblin, 2014; Sonalkar et al., 2017; Upadhyay et al., 2015; White et al., 2015; Wildschut et al., 2011; Woodcock, 2016; Zane et al., 2015). With this growing body of research, earlier abortion methods have been refined, discontinued, and new approaches have been developed (Chen and Creinin, 2015; Jatlaoui et al., 2016; Lichtenberg and Paul, 2013). For example, the use of dilation and sharp curettage is now considered obsolete in most cases because safer alternatives, such as aspiration methods, have been developed (Edelman et al, 1974; Lean et al, 1976; RCOG, 2015). The use of abortion medications in the United States began in 2000 with the approval by the U.S. Food and Drug Administration (FDA) of the drug mifepristone. In 2016, the FDA, citing extensive clinical research, updated the indications for mifepristone for medication abortion[3] up to 10 weeks' (70 days') gestation (FDA, 2016; Woodcock, 2016).

Box 1-2 describes the abortion methods currently recommended by U.S. and international medical, nursing, and other health organizations that set professional standards for reproductive health care, including the American College of Obstetricians and Gynecologists (ACOG), the Society of Family Planning, the American College of Nurse-Midwifes, the National Abortion Federation (NAF), the Royal College of Obstetricians and Gynaecologists (RCOG) (in the United Kingdom), and the World

---

[3]The terms "medication abortion" and "medical abortion" are used interchangeably in the literature.

BOX 1-2
Current Abortion Methods

Most abortions in the United States are performed in the first 13 weeks of pregnancy using either medication or aspiration methods. These and other legal abortion methods are described below. See Chapter 2 for a detailed review of the scientific evidence on the safety of each method.

- *Medication abortion* (or "medical" abortion) involves the use of medications to induce uterine contractions that expel the products of conception. The regimen, approved by the FDA for up to 70 days' (10 weeks') gestation, uses 200 mg of mifepristone followed by 800 mcg of misoprostol 24 to 48 hours later.
- *Aspiration abortion* (also referred to as surgical abortion or suction curettage) is used up to 14 to 16 weeks' gestation. A hollow curette (tube) is inserted into the uterus. At the other end of the curette, a hand-held syringe or an electric device is applied to create suction and empty the uterus.
- *Dilation and evacuation (D&E) abortion* is usually performed starting at 14 weeks' gestation. The procedure involves cervical preparation with osmotic dilators and/or medications, followed by suction and/or forceps extraction to empty the uterus. Ultrasound guidance is often used.
- *Induction abortion* (also referred to as "medical" abortion) involves the use of medications to induce labor and delivery of the fetus. The most effective regimens use a combination of mifepristone and misoprostol.

NOTE: Gestation is counted from the first day of the last menstrual period.
SOURCES: Jones and Jerman, 2017a; NAF, 2017; RCOG, 2011; WHO, 2012.

Health Organization (ACNM, 2011, 2016; ACOG, 2013, 2014; Costescu et al., 2016; Lichtenberg and Paul, 2013; NAF, 2017; RCOG, 2011; WHO, 2014).

A Continuum of Care

The committee views abortion care as a continuum of services, as illustrated in Figure 1-1. For purposes of this study, it begins when a woman, who has decided to terminate a pregnancy, contacts or visits a provider seeking an abortion. The first, preabortion phase of care includes an initial clinical assessment of the woman's overall health (e.g., physical examination, pregnancy determination, weeks of gestation, and laboratory and other testing as needed); communication of information on the risks and benefits of alternative abortion procedures and pain management options; discussion of the patient's preferences based on desired anesthesia and weeks of gestation; discussion of postabortion contraceptive options if desired; counseling

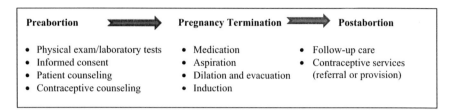

FIGURE 1-1 Continuum of abortion care.

and referral to services (if needed); and final decision making and informed consent. The next phases in the continuum are the abortion procedure itself and postabortion care, including appropriate follow-up care and provision of contraceptives (for women who opt for them).

A Note on Terminology

Important clinical terms that describe pregnancy and abortion lack consistent definition. The committee tried to be as precise as possible to avoid misinterpreting or miscommunicating the research evidence, clinical practice guidelines, and other relevant sources of information with potentially significant clinical implications. Note that this report follows Grimes and Stuart's (2010) recommendation that weeks' gestation be quantified using cardinal numbers (1, 2, 3...) rather than ordinal numbers (1st, 2nd, 3rd...). It is important to note, however, that these two numbering conventions are sometimes used interchangeably in the research literature despite having different meanings. For example, a woman who is 6 weeks pregnant has *completed* 6 weeks of pregnancy: she is in her 7th (not 6th) week of pregnancy.

This report also avoids using the term "trimester" where possible because completed weeks' or days' gestation is a more precise designation, and the clinical appropriateness of abortion methods does not align with specific trimesters.

Although the literature typically classifies the method of abortion as either "medical" or "surgical" abortion, the committee decided to specify methods more precisely by using the terminology defined in Box 1-2. The term "surgical abortion" is often used by others as a catchall category that includes a variety of procedures, ranging from an aspiration to a dilation and evacuation (D&E) procedure involving sharp surgical and other instrumentation as well as deeper levels of sedation. This report avoids describing abortion procedures as "surgical" so as to characterize a method more accurately as either an aspiration or D&E. As noted in Box 1-2, the term "induction abortion" is used to distinguish later abortions that use a medication regimen from medication abortions performed before 10 weeks' gestation.

See Appendix B for a glossary of the technical terms used in this report.

Regulation of Abortion Services

Abortion is among the most regulated medical procedures in the nation (Jones et al., 2010; Nash et al., 2017). While a comprehensive legal analysis of abortion regulation is beyond the scope of this report, the committee agreed that it should consider how abortion's unique regulatory environment relates to the safety and quality of abortion care.

In addition to the federal, state, and local rules and policies governing all medical services, numerous abortion-specific federal[4] and state laws and regulations affect the delivery of abortion services. Table 1-1 lists the abortion-specific regulations by state. The regulations range from prescribing information to be provided to women when they are counseled and setting mandatory waiting periods between counseling and the abortion procedure to those that define the clinical qualifications of abortion providers, the types of procedures they are permitted to perform, and detailed facility standards for abortion services. In addition, many states place limitations on the circumstances under which private health insurance and Medicaid can be used to pay for abortions, limiting coverage to pregnancies resulting from rape or incest or posing a medical threat to the pregnant woman's life. Other policies prevent facilities that receive state funds from providing abortion services[5] or place restrictions on the availability of services based on the gestation of the fetus that are narrower than those established under federal law (Guttmacher Institute, 2017h).

Trends and Demographics

National- and state-level abortion statistics come from two primary sources: the Centers for Disease Control and Prevention's (CDC's) Abortion

---

[4]Hyde Amendment (P.L. 94-439, 1976); Department of Defense Appropriations Act (P.L. 95-457, 1978); Peace Corps Provision and Foreign Assistance and Related Programs Appropriations Act (P.L. 95-481, 1978); Pregnancy Discrimination Act (P.L. 95-555, 1977); Department of the Treasury and Postal Service Appropriations Act (P.L. 98-151, 1983); FY1987 Continuing Resolution (P.L. 99-591, 1986); Dornan Amendment (P.L. 100-462, 1988); Partial-Birth Abortion Ban (P.L. 108-105, 2003); Weldon Amendment (P.L. 108-199, 2004); Patient Protection and Affordable Care Act (P.L. 111-148 as amended by P.L. 111-152, 2010).

[5]Personal communication, O. Cappello, Guttmacher Institute, August 4, 2017: AZ § 15-1630, GA § 20-2-773; KS § 65-6733 and § 76-3308; KY § 311.800; LA RS § 40:1299 and RS § 4 0.1061; MO § 188.210 and § 188.215; MS § 41-41-91; ND § 14-02.3-04; OH § 5101.57; OK 63 § 1-741.1; PA 18 § 3215; TX § 285.202.

TABLE 1-1 Overview of State Abortion-Specific Regulations That May Impact Safety and Quality, as of September 1, 2017

Type of Regulation[a]	States	Number of States
An ultrasound must be performed before all abortions, regardless of method	AL, AZ, FL, IA, IN, KS, LA, MS, NC, OH, OK, TX, VA, WI	14
Clinicians providing medication abortions must be in the physical presence of the patient when she takes the medication	AL, AR, AZ, IN, KS, LA, MI, MO, MS, NC, ND, NE, OK, SC, SD, TN, TX, WI, WV	19
Women must receive counseling before an abortion is performed	AL, AK, AR, AZ, CA,[b] CT,[b] FL, GA, IA, ID, IN, KS, KY, LA, ME,[b] MI, MN, MO, MS, NC, ND, NE, NV,[b] OH, OK, PA, RI,[b] SC, SD, TN, TX, UT, VA, WI, WV	35
Abortion patients are offered or given inaccurate or misleading information (verbally or in writing) on[c]		
• Reversing medication abortion	AR, SD, UT	3
• Risks to future fertility	AZ, KS, NC, NE, SD, TX	6
• Possible link to breast cancer	AK, KS, MS, OK, TX	5
• Long-term mental health consequences	ID, KS, LA, MI, NC, ND, NE, OK, SD, TX, UT, WV	12
All methods of abortion are subject to a mandatory waiting period between counseling and procedure		
• 18 hours	IN	1
• 24 hours	AZ, GA, ID, KS, KY, MI, MN, MS, ND, NE, OH, PA, SC, TX, VA, WI, WV	17
• 48 hours	AL, AR, TN	3
• 72 hours	MO, NC, OK, SD, UT	5
Preabortion counseling must be in person, necessitating two visits to the facility	AR, AZ, IN, KY, LA, MO, MS, OH, SD, TN, TX,[d] UT,[e] VA, WI	14

continued

TABLE 1-1 Continued

Type of Regulation[a]	States	Number of States
All abortions, regardless of method, must be performed by a licensed physician	AL, AK, AR, AZ, DE, FL, GA, IA, ID, IN, KS, KY, LA, MD, ME, MI, MN, MO, MS, NC, ND, NE, NV, OH, OK, PA, SC, SD, TN, TX, UT, VA, WI, WY	34
Clinicians performing any type of abortion procedures must have hospital admitting privileges or an agreement with a local hospital to transfer patients if needed	AL, AZ, IN, LA, MS, ND, OK, SC, TX, UT	10
Abortion facilities must have an agreement with a local hospital to transfer patients if needed	FL, KY, MI, NC, OH, PA, TN, WI	8
All abortions, regardless of method, must be performed in a facility that meets the structural standards typical of ambulatory surgical centers	AL, AR, AZ, IN, KY, LA, MI, MO, MS, NC, OH, OK, PA, RI, SC, SD, UT	17
Procedure room size, corridor width, or maximum distance to a hospital is specified	AL, AR, AZ,[f] FL, IN, LA, MI, MS, ND, NE, OH, OK, PA, SC, SD, UT	16
Public funding of abortions is limited to pregnancies resulting from rape or incest or when the woman's life is endangered[g]	AL, AR, CO, DC, DE, FL, GA, IA, ID, IN, KS, KY, LA, ME, MI, MO, MS, NC, ND, NE, NH, NV, OH, OK, PA, RI, SC, SD, TN, TX, UT, VA, WI, WY	34
Insurance coverage of abortion is restricted in all private insurance plans written in the state, including those offered through health insurance exchanges established under the federal health care reform law[h]	ID, IN, KS, KY, MI, MO, ND, NE, OK, TX, UT	11
Insurance coverage of abortion is restricted in plans offered through a health insurance exchange[h]	AL, AR, AZ, FL, GA, ID, IN, KS, KY, LA, MI, MO, MS, NC, ND, NE, OH, OK, PA, SC, SD, TN, TX, UT, VA, WI	26

TABLE 1-1 Continued

Type of Regulation[a]	States	Number of States
No abortions may be performed after a specified number of weeks' gestation unless the woman's life or health is endangered		
• Not after 20–22 weeks	AL, AR, GA, IA, IN, KS, KY, LA, MS, NC, ND, NE, OH, OK, SC, SD, TX, WI, WV	19
• Not at 24 weeks and after	FL, MA, NV, NY, PA, RI, VA	7
Dilation and evacuation (D&E) abortions are banned except in cases of life endangerment or severe physical health risk	MS, WV	2
Abortions cannot be performed in publicly funded facilities	AZ, GA, KS, KY, LA, MO, MS, ND, OH, OK, PA, TX	12

[a]Excludes laws or regulations permanently or temporarily enjoined pending a court decision.

[b]States have abortion-specific requirements generally following the established principles of informed consent.

[c]The content of informed consent materials is specified in state law or developed by the state department of health.

[d]In-person counseling is not required for women who live more than 100 miles from an abortion provider.

[e]Counseling requirement is waived if the pregnancy is the result of rape or incest or the patient is younger than 15.

[f]Maximum distance requirement does not apply to medication abortions.

[g]Some states also exempt women whose physical health is at severe risk and/or in cases of fetal impairment.

[h]Some states have exceptions for pregnancies resulting from rape or incest, pregnancies that severely threaten women's physical health or endanger their life, and/or in cases of fetal impairment.

SOURCES: Guttmacher Institute, 2017b,c,d,e,f,g,h,i, 2018b.

Surveillance System and the Guttmacher Institute's Abortion Provider Census (Jatlaoui et al., 2016; Jerman et al., 2016; Jones and Kavanaugh, 2011; Pazol et al., 2015). Both of these sources provide estimates of the number and rate of abortions, the use of different abortion methods, the characteristics of women who have abortions, and other related statistics. However, both sources have limitations.

The CDC system is a voluntary, state-reported system;[6,7] three states (California, Maryland, and New Hampshire) do not provide information (CDC, 2017). The Guttmacher census, also voluntary, solicits information from all known abortion providers throughout the United States, including in the states that do not submit information to the CDC surveillance system. For 2014, the latest year reported by Guttmacher,[8] information was obtained directly from 58 percent of abortion providers, and data for nonrespondents were imputed (Jones and Jerman, 2017a). The CDC's latest report, for abortions in 2013, includes approximately 70 percent of the abortions reported by the Guttmacher Institute for that year (Jatlaoui et al., 2016).

Both data collection systems report descriptive statistics on women who have abortions and the types of abortion provided, although they define demographic variables and procedure types differently. Nevertheless, in the aggregate, the trends in abortion utilization reported by the CDC and Guttmacher closely mirror each other—indicating decreasing rates of abortion, an increasing proportion of medication abortions, and the vast majority of abortions (90 percent) occurring by 13 weeks' gestation (see Figures 1-2 and 1-3) (Jatlaoui et al., 2016; Jones and Jerman, 2017a).[9] Both data sources are used in this chapter's brief review of trends in abortions and throughout the report.

Trends in the Number and Rate of Abortions

The number and rate of abortions have changed considerably during the decades following national legalization in 1973. In the immediate years after

---

[6]In most states, hospitals, facilities, and physicians are required by law to report abortion data to a central health agency. These agencies submit the aggregate utilization data to the CDC (Guttmacher Institute, 2018a).

[7]New York City and the District of Columbia also report data to the CDC.

[8]Guttmacher researchers estimate that the census undercounts the number of abortions performed in the United States by about 5 percent (i.e., 51,725 abortions provided by 2,069 obstetrician/gynecologist [OB/GYN] physicians). The estimate is based on a survey of a random sample of OB/GYN physicians. The survey did not include other physician specialties and other types of clinicians.

[9]A full-term pregnancy is 40 weeks.

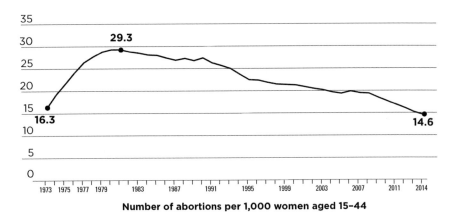

FIGURE 1-2 Abortion rate, United States, 1973–2014.
SOURCE: Guttmacher Institute, 2017a. Used with permission.

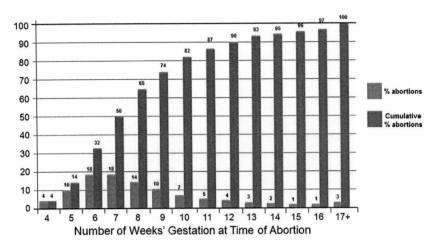

FIGURE 1-3 Percentage and cumulative percentage of outpatient abortions by weeks' gestation, 2014–2015.
NOTE: n = 8,105.
SOURCE: Adapted from Jones and Jerman, 2017b.

national legalization, both the number and rate[10] of legal abortions steadily increased (Bracken et al., 1982; Guttmacher Institute, 2017a; Pazol et al., 2015; Strauss et al., 2007) (see Figure 1-2). The abortion rate peaked in the

---

[10]Reported abortion rates are for females aged 15 to 44.

1980s, and the trend then reversed, a decline that has continued for more than three decades (Guttmacher Institute, 2017a; Jones and Kavanaugh, 2011; Pazol et al., 2015; Strauss et al., 2007). Between 1980 and 2014, the abortion rate among U.S. women fell by more than half, from 29.3 to 14.6 per 1,000 women (Finer and Henshaw, 2003; Guttmacher Institute, 2017a; Jones and Jerman, 2017a) (see Figure 1-2). In 2014, the most recent year for which data are available, the aggregate number of abortions reached a low of 926,190 after peaking at nearly 1.6 million in 1990 (Finer and Henshaw, 2003; Jones and Jerman, 2017a). The reason for the decline is not fully understood but has been attributed to several factors, including the increasing use of contraceptives, especially long-acting methods (e.g., intrauterine devices and implants); historic declines in the rate of unintended pregnancy; and increasing numbers of state regulations resulting in limited access to abortion services (Finer and Zolna, 2016; Jerman et al., 2017; Jones and Jerman, 2017a; Kost, 2015; Strauss et al., 2007).

Weeks' Gestation

Length of gestation—measured as the amount of time since the first day of the last menstrual period—is the primary factor in deciding what abortion procedure is most appropriate (ACOG, 2014). Since national legalization, most abortions in the United States have been performed in early pregnancy ($\leq$13 weeks) (Cates et al., 2000; CDC, 1983; Elam-Evans et al., 2003; Jatlaoui et al., 2016; Jones and Jerman, 2017a; Koonin and Smith, 1993; Lawson et al., 1989; Pazol et al., 2015; Strauss et al., 2007). CDC surveillance reports indicate that since at least 1992 (when detailed data on early abortions were first collected), the vast majority of abortions in the United States were early-gestation procedures (Jatlaoui et al., 2016; Strauss et al., 2007); this was the case for approximately 92 percent of all abortions in 2013 (Jatlaoui et al., 2016). With such technological advances as highly sensitive pregnancy tests and medication abortion, procedures are being performed at increasingly earlier gestational stages. According to the CDC, the percentage of early abortions performed $\leq$6 weeks' gestation increased by 16 percent from 2004 to 2013 (Jatlaoui et al., 2016); in 2013, 38 percent of early abortions occurred $\leq$6 weeks (Jatlaoui et al., 2016). The proportion of early-gestation abortions occurring $\leq$6 weeks is expected to increase even further as the use of medication abortions becomes more widespread (Jones and Boonstra, 2016; Pazol et al., 2012).

Figure 1-3 shows the proportion of abortions in nonhospital settings by weeks' gestation in 2014 (Jones and Jerman, 2017a).

Abortion Methods

Aspiration is the abortion method most commonly used in the United States, accounting for almost 68 percent of all abortions performed in 2013 (Jatlaoui et al., 2016).[11] Its use, however, is likely to decline as the use of medication abortion increases. The percentage of abortions performed by the medication method rose an estimated 110 percent between 2004 and 2013, from 10.6 to 22.3 percent (Jatlaoui et al., 2016). In 2014, approximately 45 percent of abortions performed up to 9 weeks' gestation were medication abortions, up from 36 percent in 2011 (Jones and Jerman, 2017a).

Fewer than 9 percent of abortions are performed after 13 weeks' gestation; most of these are D&E procedures (Jatlaoui et al., 2016). Induction abortion is the most infrequently used of all abortion methods, accounting for approximately 2 percent of all abortions at 14 weeks' gestation or later in 2013 (Jatlaoui et al., 2016).

Characteristics of Women Who Have Abortions

The most detailed sociodemographic statistics on women who have had an abortion in the United States are provided by the Guttmacher Institute's Abortion Patient Survey. Respondents to the 2014/2015 survey included more than 8,000 women who had had an abortion in 1 of 87 outpatient (nonhospital) facilities across the United States in 2014 (Jerman et al., 2016; Jones and Jerman, 2017b).[12] Table 1-2 provides selected findings from this survey. Although women who had an abortion in a hospital setting are excluded from these statistics, the data represent an estimated 95 percent of all abortions provided (see Figure 1-3).

The Guttmacher survey found that most women who had had an abortion were under age 30 (72 percent) and were unmarried (86 percent) (Jones and Jerman, 2017b). Women seeking an abortion were far more likely to be poor or low-income: the household income of 49 percent was below the federal poverty level (FPL), and that of 26 percent was 100 to 199 percent of the FPL (Jerman et al., 2016). In comparison, the

---

[11]CDC surveillance reports use the catchall category of "curettage" to refer to nonmedical abortion methods. The committee assumed that the CDC's curettage estimates before 13 weeks' gestation refer to aspiration procedures and that its curettage estimates after 13 weeks' gestation referred to D&E procedures.

[12]Participating facilities were randomly selected and excluded hospitals. All other types of facilities were included if they had provided at least 30 abortions in 2011 (Jerman et al., 2016). Jerman and colleagues report that logistical challenges precluded including hospital patients in the survey. The researchers believe that the exclusion of hospitals did not bias the survey sample, noting that hospitals accounted for only 4 percent of all abortions in 2011.

TABLE 1-2 Characteristics of Women Who Had an Abortion in an Outpatient Setting in 2014, by Percent

Characteristic	Percent
Age (a)	
<15–17	3.6
18–19	8.2
20–24	33.6
25–29	26.3
30–34	16.0
35+	12.2
Race/Ethnicity (a)	
Asian/Pacific Islander	4.7
Black	24.8
Hispanic	24.5
Multiracial	4.5
Other	2.5
White	39.0
Prior Pregnancies (a)	
No prior pregnancies	29.2
Prior birth only	26.0
Prior abortion only	11.7
Prior birth and abortion	33.1
Prior Births (b)	
None	40.7
1	26.2
2+	33.1
Education (a)	
Not a high school graduate	12.2
High school graduate or GED	29.0
Some college or associates degree	39.2
College graduate	19.7
Family Income as a Percentage of Federal Poverty Level (b)	
<100	49.3
100–199	25.7
≥200	25.0
Payment Method (a)	
Private insurance	14.1
Medicaid	21.9
Financial assistance	13.2
Out of pocket	45.4
Other/unknown	5.4

NOTE: Percentages may not sum to 100 because of rounding.
SOURCES: (a) Jones and Jerman, 2017b (n = 8,098); (b) Jerman et al., 2016 (n = 8,380).

corresponding percentages among all women aged 15 to 49 are 16 and 18 percent.[13] Women who had had an abortion were also more likely to be women of color[14] (61.0 percent); overall, half of women who had had an abortion were either black (24.8 percent) or Hispanic (24.5 percent) (Jones and Jerman, 2017b). This distribution is similar to the racial and ethnic distribution of women with household income below 200 percent of the FPL, 49 percent of whom are either black (20 percent) or Hispanic (29 percent).[15] Poor women and women of color are also more likely than others to experience an unintended pregnancy (Finer and Henshaw, 2006; Finer et al., 2006; Jones and Kavanaugh, 2011).

Many women who have an abortion have previously experienced pregnancy or childbirth. Among respondents to the Guttmacher survey, 59.3 percent had given birth at least once, and 44.8 percent had had a prior abortion (Jerman et al., 2016; Jones and Jerman, 2017b).

While precise estimates of health insurance coverage of abortion are not available, numerous regulations limit coverage. As noted in Table 1-1, 33 states prohibit public payers from paying for abortions and other states have laws that either prohibit health insurance exchange plans (25 states) or private insurance plans (11 states) sold in the state from covering or paying for abortions, with few exceptions.[16] In the Guttmacher survey, only 14 percent of respondents had paid for the procedure using private insurance coverage, and despite the disproportionately high rate of poverty and low income among those who had had an abortion, only 22 percent reported that Medicaid was the method of payment for their abortion. In 2015, 39 percent of the 25 million women lived in households that earned less than 200 percent of the FPL in the United States were enrolled in Medicaid, and 36 percent had private insurance (Ranji et al., 2017).

Number of Clinics Providing Abortion Care

As noted earlier, the vast majority of abortions are performed in non-hospital settings—either an abortion clinic (59 percent) or a clinic offering a variety of medical services (36 percent) (Jones and Jerman, 2017a) (see Figure 1-4). Although hospitals account for almost 40 percent of facilities offering abortion care, they provide less than 5 percent of abortions overall.

---

[13]Calculation by the committee based on estimates from *Annual Social and Economic Supplement (ASEC) to the Current Population Survey (CPS)*.

[14]Includes all nonwhite race and ethnicity categories in Table 1-2. Data were collected via self-administered questionnaire (Jones and Jerman, 2017b).

[15]Calculation by the committee based on estimates from *Annual Social and Economic Supplement (ASEC) to the Current Population Survey (CPS)*.

[16]Some states have exceptions for pregnancies resulting from rape or incest, pregnancies that endanger the woman's life or severely threaten her health, and in cases of fetal impairment.

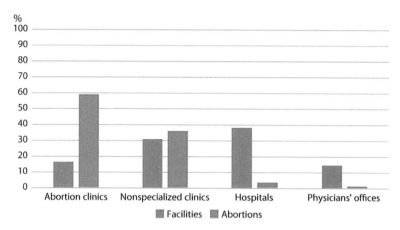

FIGURE 1-4 Percentage of abortion-providing facilities accounted for by each facility type and percentage of abortions performed in each type of facility, 2014 (n = 1,671).

NOTE: Abortion clinics are nonhospital facilities in which 50 percent or more of patient visits are for abortion services. Nonspecialized clinics are nonhospital facilities in which fewer than 50 percent of patient visits are for abortion services.

SOURCE: Jones and Jerman, 2017a.

The overall number of nonhospital facilities providing abortions—especially specialty abortion clinics—is declining. The greatest proportional decline is in states that have enacted abortion-specific regulations (Jones and Jerman, 2017a). In 2014, there were 272 abortion clinics in the United States, 17 percent fewer than in 2011. The greatest decline (26 percent) was among large clinics with annual caseloads of 1,000–4,999 patients and clinics in the Midwest (22 percent) and the South (13 percent). In 2014, approximately 39 percent of U.S. women aged 15 to 44 resided in a U.S. county without an abortion provider (90 percent of counties overall) (Jones and Jerman, 2017a). Twenty-five states have five or fewer abortion clinics; five states have one abortion clinic (Jones and Jerman, 2017a). A recent analysis[17] by Guttmacher evaluated geographic disparities in access to abortion by calculating the distance between women of reproductive age (15 to 44) and the nearest abortion-providing facility in 2014 (Bearak et al., 2017). Figure 1-5 highlights the median distance to the nearest facility by county.

---

[17]The analysis was limited to facilities that provided at least 400 abortions per year and those affiliated with Planned Parenthood that performed at least 1 abortion during the period of analysis.

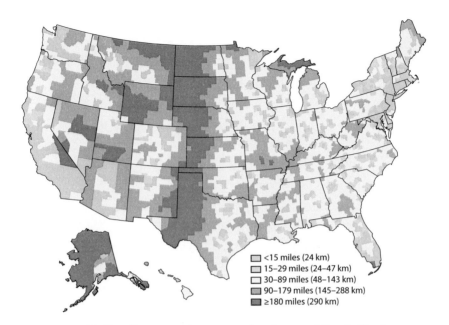

FIGURE 1-5 Median distance to the nearest abortion-providing facility by county, 2014.
NOTE: Analysis is limited to facilities that had caseloads of 400 abortions or more per year and those affiliated with Planned Parenthood that performed at least 1 abortion in the period of analysis.
SOURCE: Bearak et al., 2017.

The majority of facilities offer early medication and aspiration abortions. In 2014, 87 percent of nonhospital facilities provided early medication abortions; 23 percent of all nonhospital facilities offered this type of abortion (Jones and Jerman, 2017a). Fewer facilities offer later-gestation procedures, and availability decreases as gestation increases. In 2012, 95 percent of all abortion facilities offered abortions at 8 weeks' gestation, 72 percent at 12 weeks' gestation, 34 percent at 20 weeks' gestation, and 16 percent at 24 weeks' gestation (Jerman and Jones, 2014).

STUDY APPROACH

Conceptual Framework

The committee's approach to this study built on two foundational developments in the understanding and evaluation of the quality of health

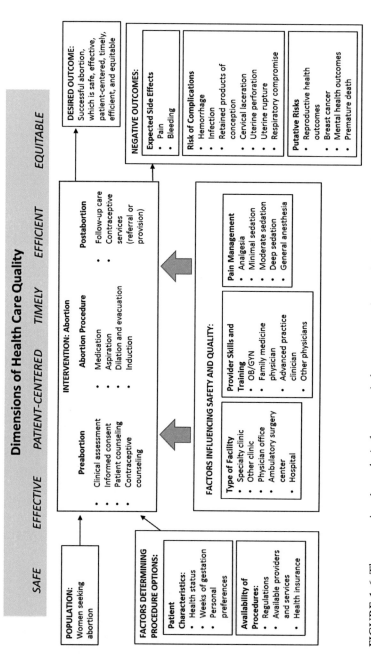

FIGURE 1-6 The committee's analytic framework for assessing the quality of abortion care.
NOTE: OB/GYN = obstetrician/gynecologist.

care services: Donabedian's (1980) structure-process-outcome framework and the IOM's (2001) six dimensions of quality health care. Figure 1-6 illustrates the committee's adaptation of these concepts for this study's assessment of abortion care in the United States.

Structure-Process-Outcome Framework

In seminal work published almost 40 years ago, Donabedian (1980) proposed that the quality of health care be assessed by examining its structure, process, and outcomes (Donabedian, 1980):

- *Structure* refers to organizational factors that may create the potential for good quality. In abortion care, such structural factors as the availability of trained staff and the characteristics of the clinical setting may ensure—or inhibit—the capacity for quality.
- *Process* refers to what is done to and for the patient. Its assessment assumes that the services patients receive should be evidence based and correlated with patients' desired outcomes—for example, an early and complete abortion for women who wish to terminate an unintended pregnancy.
- *Outcomes* are the end results of care—the effects of the intervention on the health and well-being of the patient. Does the procedure achieve its objective? Does it lead to serious health risks in the short or long term?

Six Dimensions of Health Care Quality

The landmark IOM report *Crossing the Quality Chasm: A New Health System for the 21st Century* (IOM, 2001) identifies six dimensions of health care quality—safety, effectiveness, patient-centeredness, timeliness, efficiency, and equity. The articulation of these six dimensions has guided public and private efforts to improve U.S. health care delivery at the local, state, and national levels since that report was published (AHRQ, 2016).

In addition, as with other health care services, women should expect that the abortion care they receive meets well-established standards for objectivity, transparency, and scientific rigor (IOM, 2011a,b).

Two of the IOM's six dimensions—safety and effectiveness—are particularly salient to the present study. Assessing both involves making relative judgments. There are no universally agreed-upon thresholds for defining care as "safe" versus "unsafe" or "effective" versus "not effective," and decisions about safety and effectiveness have a great deal to do with the context of the clinical scenario. Thus, the committee's frame of reference for evaluating safety, effectiveness, and other quality domains is of necessity a relative one—one that entails not only comparing the alternative abortion methods but also comparing these methods with other health care services and with risks associated with not achieving the desired outcome.

Safety—avoiding injury to patients—is often assessed by measuring the incidence and severity of complications and other adverse events associated with receiving a specific procedure. If infrequent, a complication may be characterized as "rare"—a term that lacks consistent definition. In this report, "rare" is used to describe outcomes that affect fewer than 1 percent of patients. Complications are considered "serious" if they result in a blood transfusion, surgery, or hospitalization.

Note also that the term "effectiveness" is used differently in this report depending on the context. As noted in Box 1-3, effectiveness as an attribute of quality refers to providing services based on scientific knowledge to all who could benefit and refraining from providing services to those not likely to benefit (avoiding underuse and overuse, respectively). Elsewhere in this report, effectiveness denotes the clinical effectiveness of a procedure, that

---

BOX 1-3
The Six Dimensions of Health Care Quality

Crossing the Quality Chasm: A New Health System for the 21st Century

1. Safety—avoiding injuries to patients from the care that is intended to help them.

2. Effectiveness—providing services based on scientific knowledge to all who could benefit and refraining from providing services to those not likely to benefit (avoiding underuse and overuse, respectively).

3. Patient-centeredness—providing care that is respectful of and responsive to individual patient preferences, needs, and values and ensuring that patient values guide all clinical decisions.

4. Timeliness—reducing waits and sometimes harmful delays for both those who receive and those who give care.

5. Efficiency—avoiding waste, including waste of equipment, supplies, ideas, and energy.

6. Equity—providing care that does not vary in quality because of personal characteristics such as gender, ethnicity, geographic location, and socioeconomic status.

SOURCE: Excerpted from IOM, 2001, p. 6.

is, the successful completion of an abortion without the need for a follow-up aspiration.

Finding and Assessing the Evidence

The committee deliberated during four in-person meetings and numerous teleconferences between January 2017 and December 2017. On March 24, 2017, the committee hosted a public workshop at the Keck Center of the National Academies of Sciences, Engineering, and Medicine in Washington, DC. The workshop included presentations from three speakers on topics related to facility standards and the safety of outpatient procedures. Appendix C contains the workshop agenda.

Several committee workgroups were formed to find and assess the quality of the available evidence and to draft summary materials for the full committee's review. The workgroups conducted in-depth reviews of the epidemiology of abortions, including rates of complications and mortality, the safety and effectiveness of alternative abortion methods, professional standards and methods for performing all aspects of abortion care (as described in Figure 1-1), the short- and long-term physical and mental health effects of having an abortion; and the safety and quality implications of abortion-specific regulations on abortion.

The committee focused on finding reliable, scientific information reflecting contemporary U.S. abortion practices. An extensive body of research on abortion has been conducted outside the United States. A substantial proportion of this literature concerns the delivery of abortion care in countries where socioeconomic conditions, culture, population health, health care resources, and/or the health care system are markedly different from their U.S. counterparts. Studies from other countries were excluded from this review if the committee judged those factors to be relevant to the health outcomes being assessed.

The committee considered evidence from randomized controlled trials comparing two or more approaches to abortion care; systematic reviews; meta-analyses; retrospective cohort studies, case control studies, and other types of observational studies; and patient and provider surveys (see Box 1-4).

An extensive literature documents the biases common in published research on the effectiveness of health care services (Altman et al., 2001; Glasziou et al., 2008; Hopewell et al., 2008; Ioannidis et al., 2004; IOM, 2011a,b; Plint et al., 2006; Sackett, 1979; von Elm et al., 2007). Thus, the committee prioritized the available research according to conventional principles of evidence-based medicine intended to reduce the risk of bias in a study's conclusions, such as how subjects were allocated to different types of abortion care, the comparability of study populations, controls

---

BOX 1-4
Types of Research Reviewed for This Study

The following types of experimental and observational research on the outcomes of abortion care were reviewed for this study.

Experimental Studies

- **Controlled trials** are experimental studies in which an experimental group receives the intervention of interest while one or more comparison groups receive an active comparator, a placebo, no intervention, or the usual standard of care, and the outcomes are compared. In a randomized controlled trial (RCT), the participants are randomly allocated to the experimental group or the comparison group(s).
- **Systematic reviews** are scientific investigations focused on a specific question and use explicit, planned scientific methods to identify, select, assess, and summarize the findings of similar but separate studies. They may or may not include a quantitative synthesis (meta-analysis) of the results from separate studies.
- A **meta-analysis** is a systematic review that uses statistical methods to combine quantitatively the results of similar studies in an attempt to allow inferences to be drawn from the sample of studies and applied to the population of interest.

Observational Studies

- In **cohort studies**, groups of exposed individuals (e.g., women having had an abortion in their first pregnancy) and groups of unexposed individuals (e.g., women whose first pregnancy was a delivery) are monitored over time and compared with respect to an outcome of interest (e.g., future fertility). Cohort studies can be either prospective or retrospective.
- **Case control studies** compare one group of persons with a certain disease, chronic condition, or type of injury (case patients) and another group of persons without that health problem (control subjects) to identify differences in exposures, behaviors, and other characteristics for the purpose of determining and quantifying associations, testing hypotheses, and understanding causes.

SOURCE: IOM, 2011b.

---

for confounding factors, how outcome assessments were conducted, the completeness of outcome reporting, the representativeness of the study population compared with the general U.S. population, and the degree to which statistical analyses helped reduce bias (IOM, 2011b). Applying these principles is particularly important with respect to understanding abortion's long-term health effects, an area in which the relevant literature is vulnerable to bias (as discussed in Chapter 4).

The committee's literature search strategy is described in Appendix D.

ORGANIZATION OF THE REPORT

Chapter 2 of this report describes the continuum of abortion care including current abortion methods (question 1 in the committee's statement of task [Box 1-1]); reviews the evidence on factors affecting their safety and quality, including expected side effects and possible complications (questions 2 and 3), necessary safeguards to manage medical emergencies (question 6), and provision of pain management (question 7); and presents the evidence on the types of facilities or facility factors necessary to provide safe and effective abortion care (question 4).

Chapter 3 summarizes the clinical skills that are integral to safe and high-quality abortion care according to the recommendations of leading national professional organizations and abortion training curricula (question 5).

Chapter 4 reviews research examining the long-term health effects of undergoing an abortion (question 2).

Finally, Chapter 5 presents the committee's conclusions regarding the findings presented in the previous chapters, responding to each of the questions posed in the statement of task. Findings are statements of scientific evidence. The report's conclusions are the committee's inferences, interpretations, or generalizations drawn from the evidence.

REFERENCES

ACNM (American College of Nurse-Midwives). 2011. *Position statement: Reproductive health choices.* http://www.midwife.org/ACNM/files/ACNMLibraryData/UPLOADFILE NAME/000000000087/Reproductive_Choices.pdf (accessed August 1, 2017).
ACNM. 2016. *Position statement: Access to comprehensive sexual and reproductive health care services.* http://www.midwife.org/ACNM/files/ACNMLibraryData/UPLOADFILE NAME/000000000087/Access-to-Comprehensive-Sexual-and-Reproductive-Health-Care-Services-FINAL-04-12-17.pdf (accessed August 1, 2017).
ACOG (American College of Obstetricians and Gynecologists). 2013. Practice Bulletin No. 135: Second-trimester abortion. *Obstetrics & Gynecology* 121(6):1394–1406.
ACOG. 2014. Practice Bulletin No. 143: Medical management of first-trimester abortion (reaffirmed). *Obstetrics & Gynecology* 123(3):676–692.
AHRQ (Agency for Healthcare Research and Quality). 2016. *The six domains of health care quality.* https://www.ahrq.gov/professionals/quality-patient-safety/talkingquality/create/sixdomains.html (accessed May 3, 2017).
Altman, D. G., K. F. Schulz, D. Moher, M. Egger, F. Davidoff, D. Elbourne, P. C. Gøtzsche, and T. Lang. 2001. The revised CONSORT statement for reporting randomized trials: Explanation and elaboration. *Annals of Internal Medicine* 134(8):663–694.

Ashok, P. W., A. Templeton, P. T. Wagaarachchi, and G. M. Flett. 2004. Midtrimester medical termination of pregnancy: A review of 1002 consecutive cases. *Contraception* 69(1):51–58.

Autry, A. M., E. C. Hayes, G. F. Jacobson, and R. S. Kirby. 2002. A comparison of medical induction and dilation and evacuation for second-trimester abortion. *American Journal of Obstetrics and Gynecology* 187(2):393–397.

Bartlett, L. A., C. J. Berg, H. B. Shulman, S. B. Zane, C. A. Green, S. Whitehead, and H. K. Atrash. 2004. Risk factors for legal induced abortion-related mortality in the United States. *Obstetrics & Gynecology* 103(4):729–737.

Bearak, J. M., K. L. Burke, and R. K. Jones. 2017. Disparities and change over time in distance women would need to travel to have an abortion in the USA: A spatial analysis. *The Lancet Public Health* 2(11):e493–e500.

Borgatta, L. 2011. *Labor induction termination of pregnancy. Global library for women's medicine.* https://www.glowm.com/section_view/heading/Labor%20Induction%20Termination%20of%20Pregnancy/item/443 (accessed September 13, 2017).

Borkowski, L., J. Strasser, A. Allina, and S. Wood. 2015. *Medication abortion. Overview of research & policy in the United States.* http://publichealth.gwu.edu/sites/default/files/Medication_Abortion_white_paper.pdf (accessed January 25, 2017).

Bracken, M. B., D. H. Freeman, Jr., and K. Hellenbrand. 1982. Hospitalization for medical-legal and other abortions in the United States 1970–1977. *American Journal of Public Health* 72(1):30–37.

Bryant, A. G., D. A. Grimes, J. M. Garrett, and G. S. Stuart. 2011. Second-trimester abortion for fetal anomalies or fetal death: Labor induction compared with dilation and evacuation. *Obstetrics & Gynecology* 117(4):788–792.

Cates, Jr., W., K. F. Schulz, D. A. Grimes, A. J. Horowitz, F. A. Lyon, F. H. Kravitz, and M. J. Frisch. 1982. Dilatation and evacuation procedures and second-trimester abortions. The role of physician skill and hospital setting. *Journal of the American medical Association* 248(5):559–563.

Cates, Jr., W., D. A. Grimes, and K. F. Schulz. 2000. Abortion surveillance at CDC: Creating public health light out of political heat. *American Journal of Preventive Medicine* 19(1, Suppl. 1):12–17.

CDC (Centers for Disease Control and Prevention). 1983. Surveillance summary abortion surveillance: Preliminary analysis, 1979–1980—United States. *MMWR Weekly* 32(5): 62–64. https://www.cdc.gov/mmwr/preview/mmwrhtml/00001243.htm (accessed September 18, 2017).

CDC. 2017. *CDC's abortion surveillance system FAQs.* https://www.cdc.gov/reproductivehealth/data_stats/abortion.htm (accessed June 22, 2017).

Chen, M. J., and M. D. Creinin. 2015. Mifepristone with buccal misoprostol for medical abortion: A systematic review. *Obstetrics & Gynecology* 126(1):12–21.

Cleland, K., M. D. Creinin, D. Nucatola, M. Nshom, and J. Trussell. 2013. Significant adverse events and outcomes after medical abortion. *Obstetrics & Gynecology* 121(1):166–171.

Costescu, D., E. Guilbert, J. Bernardin, A. Black, S. Dunn, B. Fitzsimmons, W. V. Norman, H. Pymar, J. Soon, K. Trouton, M. S. Wagner, and E. Wiebe. 2016. Medical abortion. *Journal of Obstetrics and Gynaecology Canada* 38(4):366–389.

Donabedian, A. 1980. The definition of quality and approaches to its assessment. In *Explorations in quality assessment and monitoring.* Vol. 1. Ann Arbor, MI: Health Administration Press.

Edelman, D. A., W. E. Brenner, and G. S. Berger. 1974. The effectiveness and complications of abortion by dilatation and vacuum aspiration versus dilatation and rigid metal curettage. *American Journal of Obstetrics and Gynecology* 119(4):473–480.

Elam-Evans, L. D., L. T. Strauss, J. Herndon, W. Y. Parker, S. V. Bowens, S. Zane, and C. J. Berg. 2003. Abortion surveillance—United States, 2000. *MMWR Surveillance Summaries* 52(SS-12):1–32. https://www.cdc.gov/mmwr/preview/mmwrhtml/ss5212a1.htm (accessed September 18, 2017).

FDA (U.S. Food and Drug Administration). 2016. *MIFEPREX®: Highlights* of prescribing information. https://www.accessdata.fda.gov/drugsatfda_docs/label/2016/020687s020lbl. pdf (accessed September 11, 2017).

Finer, L. B., and S. K. Henshaw. 2003. Abortion incidence and services in the United States in 2000. *Perspectives on Sexual and Reproductive Health* 35(1):6–15.

Finer, L. B., and S. K. Henshaw. 2006. Disparities in rates of unintended pregnancy in the United States, 1994 and 2001. *Perspectives on Sexual and Reproductive Health* 38(2):90–96.

Finer, L. B., and M. R. Zolna. 2016. Declines in unintended pregnancy in the United States, 2008–2011. *New England Journal of Medicine* 374(9):843–852.

Finer, L. B., L. F. Frohwirth, L. A. Dauphinee, S. Singh, and A. M. Moore. 2006. Timing of steps and reasons for delays in obtaining abortions in the United States. *Contraception* 74(4):334–344.

Frick, A. C., E. A. Drey, J. T. Diedrich, and J. E. Steinauer. 2010. Effect of prior cesarean delivery on risk of second-trimester surgical abortion complications. *Obstetrics & Gynecology* 115(4):760–764.

Gary, M. M., and D. J. Harrison. 2006. Analysis of severe adverse events related to the use of mifepristone as an abortifacient. *Annals of Pharmacotherapy* 40(2):191–197.

Glasziou, P., E. Meats, C. Heneghan, and S. Shepperd. 2008. What is missing from descriptions of treatment in trials and reviews? *British Medical Journal* 336(7659):1472–1474.

Grimes, D. A., and G. Stuart. 2010. Abortion jabberwocky: The need for better terminology. *Contraception* 81(2):93–96.

Grimes, D. A., S. M. Smith, and A. D. Witham. 2004. Mifepristone and misoprostol versus dilation and evacuation for midtrimester abortion: A pilot randomised controlled trial. *British Journal of Obstetrics & Gynaecology* 111(2):148–153.

Grossman, D., K. Blanchard, and P. Blumenthal. 2008. Complications after second trimester surgical and medical abortion. *Reproductive Health Matters* 16(31 Suppl.):173–182.

Grossman, D., K. Grindlay, T. Buchacker, K. Lane, and K. Blanchard. 2011. Effectiveness and acceptability of medical abortion provided through telemedicine. *Obstetrics & Gynecology* 118(2 Pt. 1):296–303.

Guttmacher Institute. 2017a. *Fact sheet: Induced abortion in the United States.* https://www.guttmacher.org/fact-sheet/induced-abortion-united-states (accessed November 10, 2017).

Guttmacher Institute. 2017b. *Bans on specific abortion methods used after the first trimester.* https://www.guttmacher.org/state-policy/explore/bans-specific-abortion-methods-used-after-first-trimester (accessed September 12, 2017).

Guttmacher Institute. 2017c. *Counseling and waiting periods for abortion.* https://www.guttmacher.org/state-policy/explore/counseling-and-waiting-periods-abortion (accessed September 12, 2017).

Guttmacher Institute. 2017d. *Medication abortion.* https://www.guttmacher.org/state-policy/explore/medication-abortion (accessed September 12, 2017).

Guttmacher Institute. 2017e. *An overview of abortion laws.* https://www.guttmacher.org/state-policy/explore/overview-abortion-laws (accessed September 12, 2017).

Guttmacher Institute. 2017f. *Requirements for ultrasound.* https://www.guttmacher.org/state-policy/explore/requirements-ultrasound (accessed September 12, 2017).

Guttmacher Institute. 2017g. *State funding of abortion under Medicaid.* https://www.guttmacher.org/state-policy/explore/state-funding-abortion-under-medicaid (accessed September 12, 2017).

Guttmacher Institute. 2017h. *State policies on later abortions.* https://www.guttmacher.org/state-policy/explore/state-policies-later-abortions (accessed September 12, 2017).

Guttmacher Institute. 2017i. *Targeted regulation of abortion providers.* https://www.guttmacher.org/state-policy/explore/targeted-regulation-abortion-providers (accessed September 12, 2017).

Guttmacher Institute. 2018a. *Abortion reporting requirements.* https://www.guttmacher.org/state-policy/explore/abortion-reporting-requirements (accessed January 22, 2018).

Guttmacher Institute. 2018b. *Restricting insurance coverage of abortion.* https://www.guttmacher.org/state-policy/explore/restricting-insurance-coverage-abortion (accessed January 24, 2018).

Hopewell, S., M. Clarke, D. Moher, E. Wager, P. Middleton, D. G. Altman, K. F. Schulz, and the CONSORT Group. 2008. CONSORT for reporting randomized controlled trials in journal and conference abstracts: Explanation and elaboration. *PLoS Medicine* 5(1):e20.

Ioannidis, J. P., S. J. Evans, P. C. Gøtzsche, R. T. O'Neill, D. G. Altman, K. Schulz, D. Moher, and the CONSORT Group. 2004. Better reporting of harms in randomized trials: An extension of the CONSORT statement. *Annals of Internal Medicine* 141(10):781–788.

IOM (Institute of Medicine). 1975. *Legalized abortion and the public health.* Washington, DC: National Academy Press.

IOM. 2001. *Crossing the quality chasm: A new health system for the 21st century.* Washington, DC: National Academy Press.

IOM. 2011a. *Clinical practice guidelines we can trust.* Washington, DC: The National Academies Press.

IOM. 2011b. *Finding what works in health care: Standards for systematic reviews.* Washington, DC: The National Academies Press.

Ireland, L. D., M. Gatter, and A. Y. Chen. 2015. Medical compared with surgical abortion for effective pregnancy termination in the first trimester. *Obstetrics & Gynecology* 126(1):22–28.

Jatlaoui, T. C., A. Ewing, M. G. Mandel, K. B. Simmons, D. B. Suchdev, D. J. Jamieson, and K. Pazol. 2016. Abortion surveillance—United States, 2013. *MMWR Surveillance Summaries* 65(No. SS-12):1–44.

Jerman, J., and R. K. Jones. 2014. Secondary measures of access to abortion services in the United States, 2011 and 2012: Gestational age limits, cost, and harassment. *Women's Health Issues* 24(4): e419–e424.

Jerman J., R. K. Jones, and T. Onda. 2016. *Characteristics of U.S. abortion patients in 2014 and changes since 2008.* https://www.guttmacher.org/sites/default/files/report_pdf/characteristics-us-abortion-patients-2014.pdf (accessed October 17, 2016).

Jerman, J., L. Frohwirth, M. L. Kavanaugh, and N. Blades. 2017. Barriers to abortion care and their consequences for patients traveling for services: Qualitative findings from two states. *Perspectives on Sexual and Reproductive Health* 49(2):95–102.

Jones, R. K., and H. D. Boonstra. 2016. *The public health implications of the FDA update to the medication abortion label.* New York: Guttmacher Institute. https://www.guttmacher.org/article/2016/06/public-health-implications-fda-update-medication-abortion-label (accessed October 27, 2017).

Jones, R. K., and J. Jerman. 2017a. Abortion incidence and service availability in the United States, 2014. *Perspectives on Sexual and Reproductive Health* 49(1):1–11.

Jones, R. K., and J. Jerman. 2017b. Characteristics and circumstances of U.S. women who obtain very early and second trimester abortions. *PLoS One* 12(1):e0169969.

Jones, R. K., and M. L. Kavanaugh. 2011. Changes in abortion rates between 2000 and 2008 and lifetime incidence of abortion. *Obstetrics & Gynecology* 117(6):1358–1366.

Jones, R. K., L. B. Finer, and S. Singh. 2010. *Characteristics of U.S. abortion patients, 2008.* New York: Guttmacher Institute.

Kahn, J. B., J. P. Bourne, J. D. Asher, and C. W. Tyler. 1971. Technical reports: Surveillance of abortions in hospitals in the United States, 1970. *HSMHA Health Reports* 86(5):423–430.

Kelly, T., J. Suddes, D. Howel, J. Hewison, and S. Robson. 2010. Comparing medical versus surgical termination of pregnancy at 13–20 weeks of gestation: A randomised controlled trial. *British Journal of Obstetrics & Gynaecology* 117(12): 1512–1520.

Koonin, L. M., and J. C. Smith. 1993. Abortion surveillance—United States, 1990. *MMWR Surveillance Summaries* 42(SS-6):29–57. https://www.cdc.gov/mmwr/preview/mmwrhtml/00031585.htm (accessed September 18, 2017).

Kost, K. 2015. *Unintended pregnancy rates at the state level: Estimates for 2010 and trends since 2002.* New York: Guttmacher Institute.

Kulier, R., N. Kapp, A. M. Gulmezoglu, G. J. Hofmeyr, L. Cheng, and A. Campana. 2011. Medical methods for first trimester abortion. *The Cochrane Database of Systematic Reviews* (11):CD002855.

Lawson, H. W., H. K. Atrash, A. F. Saftlas, L. M. Koonin, M. Ramick, and J. C. Smith. 1989. Abortion surveillance, United States, 1984–1985. *MMWR Surveillance Summaries* 38(SS-2):11–15. https://www.cdc.gov/Mmwr/preview/mmwrhtml/00001467.htm (accessed September 18, 2017).

Lean, T. H., D. Vengadasalam, S. Pachauri, and E. R. Miller. 1976. A comparison of D & C and vacuum aspiration for performing first trimester abortion. *International Journal of Gynecology and Obstetrics* 14(6):481–486.

Lichtenberg, E. S., and M. Paul. 2013. Surgical abortion prior to 7 weeks of gestation. *Contraception* 88(1):7–17.

Lohr, A. P., J. L. Hayes, and K. Gemzell Danielsson. 2008. Surgical versus medical methods for second trimester induced abortion. *Cochrane Database of Systematic Reviews* (1):CD006714.

Low, N., M. Mueller, H. A. Van Vliet, and N. Kapp. 2012. Perioperative antibiotics to prevent infection after first-trimester abortion. *Cochrane Database of Systematic Reviews* (3):CD005217.

Mauelshagen, A., L. C. Sadler, H. Roberts, M. Harilall, and C. M. Farquhar. 2009. Audit of short term outcomes of surgical and medical second trimester termination of pregnancy. *Reproductive Health* 6(1):16.

NAF (National Abortion Federation). 2017. *2017 Clinical policy guidelines for abortion care.* Washington, DC: NAF.

Nash, E., R. B. Gold, L. Mohammed, O. Cappello, and Z. Ansari-Thomas. 2017. *Laws affecting reproductive health and rights: State policy trends at midyear, 2017.* Washington, DC: Guttmacher Institute. https://www.guttmacher.org/article/2017/07/laws-affecting-reproductive-health-and-rights-state-policy-trends-midyear-2017 (accessed September 21, 2017).

Ngoc, N. T., T. Shochet, S. Raghavan, J. Blum, N. T. Nga, N. T. Minh, V. Q. Phan, B. Winikoff. 2011. Mifepristone and misoprostol compared with misoprostol alone for second-trimester abortion: A randomized controlled trial. *Obstetrics & Gynecology* 118(3):601–608.

Ohannessian, A., K. Baumstarck, J. Maruani, E. Cohen-Solal, P. Auquier, and A. Agostini. 2016. Mifepristone and misoprostol for cervical ripening in surgical abortion between 12 and 14 weeks of gestation: A randomized controlled trial. *European Journal of Obstetrics & Gynecology and Reproductive Biology* 201:151–155.

Pazol, K., A. A. Creanga, and S. B. Zane. 2012. Trends in use of medical abortion in the United States: Reanalysis of surveillance data from the Centers for Disease Control and Prevention, 2001–2008. *Contraception* 86(6):746–751.

Pazol, K., A. A. Creanga, and D. J. Jamieson. 2015. Abortion surveillance—United States, 2012. *Morbidity and Mortality Weekly Report* 64(SS-10):1–40.

Peterson, W. F., F. N. Berry, M. R. Grace, and C. L. Gulbranson. 1983. Second-trimester abortion by dilatation and evacuation: An analysis of 11,747 cases. *Obstetrics & Gynecology* 62(2):185–190.

Plint, A. C., D. Moher, A. Morrison, K. Schulz, D. G. Altman, C. Hill, and I. Gaboury. 2006. Does the CONSORT checklist improve the quality of reports of randomised controlled trials? A systematic review. *Medical Journal of Australia* 185(5):263–267.

Ranji, U., A. Salganicoff, L. Sobel, C. Rosenzweig, and I. Gomez. 2017. *Financing family planning services for low-income women: The role of public programs.* https://www.kff. org/womens-health-policy/issue-brief/financing-family-planning-services-for-low-income-women-the-role-of-public-programs (accessed September 9, 2017).

Raymond, E. G., C. Shannon, M. A. Weaver, and B. Winikoff. 2013. First-trimester medical abortion with mifepristone 200 mg and misoprostol: A systematic review. *Contraception* 87(1):26–37.

RCOG (Royal College of Obstetricians and Gynaecologists). 2011. The care of women requesting induced abortion (Evidence-based clinical guideline number 7). London, UK: RCOG Press. https://www.rcog.org.uk/globalassets/documents/guidelines/abortion-guideline_web_1.pdf (accessed July 27, 2017).

RCOG. 2015. Best practice in comprehensive abortion care (Best practice paper no. 2). London, UK: RCOG Press. https://www.rcog.org.uk/globalassets/documents/guidelines/best-practice-papers/best-practice-paper-2.pdf (accessed September 11, 2017).

Roblin, P. 2014. Vacuum aspiration. In *Abortion care*, edited by S. Rowlands. Cambridge, UK: Cambridge University Press.

Sackett, D. L. 1979. Bias in analytic research. *Journal of Chronic Diseases* 32(1–2):51–63.

Sonalkar, S., S. N. Ogden, L. K. Tran, and A. Y. Chen. 2017. Comparison of complications associated with induction by misoprostol versus dilation and evacuation for second-trimester abortion. *International Journal of Gynaecology & Obstetrics* 138(3):272–275.

Strauss, L. T., S. B. Gamble, W. Y. Parker, D. A. Cook, S. B. Zane, and S. Hamdan. 2007. Abortion surveillance—United States, 2004. *MMWR Surveillance Summaries* 56 (SS-12):1–33.

Upadhyay, U. D., S. Desai, V. Zlidar, T. A. Weitz, D. Grossman, P. Anderson, and D. Taylor. 2015. Incidence of emergency department visits and complications after abortion. *Obstetrics & Gynecology* 125(1):175–183.

von Elm, E., D. G. Altman, M. Egger, S. J. Pocock, P. C. Gøtzsche, and J. P. Vandenbrouke. 2007. The Strengthening the Reporting of Observational Studies in Epidemiology (STROBE) statement: Guidelines for reporting observational studies. *PLoS Medicine* 4(10):e296.

White, K., E. Carroll, and D. Grossman. 2015. Complications from first-trimester aspiration abortion: A systematic review of the literature. *Contraception* 92(5):422–438.

WHO (World Health Organization). 2012. *Safe abortion: Technical and policy guidance for health systems* (Second edition). http://apps.who.int/iris/bitstream/10665/70914/1/9789241548434_eng.pdf (accessed September 12, 2017).

WHO. 2014. *Clinical practice handbook for safe abortion.* Geneva, Switzerland: WHO Press. http://apps.who.int/iris/bitstream/10665/97415/1/9789241548717_eng.pdf?ua=1&ua=1 (accessed November 15, 2016).

Wildschut, H., M. I. Both, S. Medema, E. Thomee, M. F. Wildhagen, and N. Kapp. 2011. Medical methods for mid-trimester termination of pregnancy. *The Cochrane Database of Systematic Reviews* (1):Cd005216.

Woodcock, J. 2016. Letter from the director of the FDA Center for Drug Evaluation and Research to Donna Harrison, Gene Rudd, and Penny Young Nance. *Re: Docket No. FDA-2002-P-0364.* Silver Spring, MD: FDA.

Zane, S., A. A. Creanga, C. J. Berg, K. Pazol, D. B. Suchdev, D. J. Jamieson, and W. M. Callaghan. 2015. Abortion-related mortality in the United States: 1998–2010. *Obstetrics & Gynecology* 126(2):258–265.

2

The Safety and Quality of Current Abortion Methods

In the more than 40 years since national legalization of abortion, investigators have conducted randomized controlled trials (RCTs), large retrospective cohort studies, patient and provider surveys, systematic reviews, and other types of research on abortion care and its health effects on women, resulting in an extensive literature. The objective of this chapter is to examine this literature, focusing on the safety and effectiveness of current abortion methods and the extent to which these methods could expose women to the risk of such serious complications as the need for blood transfusion, surgery, or hospitalization. The chapter also examines whether the type of facility or method of sedation or anesthesia affects the risk of adverse outcomes. The chapter is organized as follows:

- The first section describes the clinical assessment, informed consent, patient education, and counseling that precede the abortion procedure.
- The second section addresses the initial clinical assessment.
- The next section describes current abortion methods and, for each method, reviews what is known about the procedure's effectiveness, expected side effects, and risk of complications. Note that, for the purposes of this review, efficacy or effectiveness refers to the successful completion of the abortion without the need for a follow-up aspiration.
- The fourth section turns to postabortion care.

- The fifth section examines the evidence on the use of analgesia, sedation, and anesthesia in abortion care, including its safety and implications for the site of care.
- The following section compares the mortality rates for abortion and other common outpatient procedures.
- The next section presents a brief discussion of state regulation of abortion care.
- The final, summary section reviews state regulation of abortion safety in light of the clinical evidence presented earlier in the chapter.

The committee's review emphasizes contemporary approaches to abortion care because abortion methods have been refined in response to new evidence. Some research conducted before 2000 is unlikely to reflect the outcomes of how abortions are typically performed in the United States today. As discussed below, for example, the U.S. Food and Drug Administration (FDA)-approved protocol for medication abortion was updated in 2016 based on extensive research showing improved outcomes with a revised regimen (CDER, 2016). Techniques used in aspiration procedures are also safer and more effective than in the past. Sharp metal curettes, once commonly used, are considered obsolete by many professional groups, and their use is no longer recommended for abortion because of the increased (albeit rare) risk of injury (NAF, 2017a; RCOG, 2011, 2015; Roblin, 2014; SFP, 2013; WHO, 2012). New approaches to cervical preparation and the use of ultrasound guidance have also improved abortion safety (Darney and Sweet, 1989; SFP, 2013).

This chapter draws primarily on the scientific literature but also includes the recommendations (i.e., clinical practice guidelines and best practices) of professional groups that provide obstetrical and gynecological care or are concerned with the quality of abortion services. Appendix D summarizes the literature search strategies the committee used to identify the relevant evidence, while Table 2-1 describes the sources of the clinical guidelines cited throughout this report.

PREABORTION CARE

When women seek an abortion, they present with a variety of experiences and needs (Moore et al., 2011; Zurek et al., 2015). Patient-centeredness—a fundamental attribute of quality health care—means "providing care that is respectful of and responsive to individual patient preferences, needs, and values and ensuring that patient values guide all clinical decisions" (IOM, 2001, p. 6). Thus, when women seek an abortion, they should have the opportunity to discuss their questions and concerns and receive support in their decision making. They should also

TABLE 2-1 Selected Organizations That Issue Clinical Guidelines on Abortion Care

American College of Obstetricians and Gynecologists (ACOG)	A professional membership organization of obstetricians and gynecologists. ACOG produces clinical guidelines and other educational materials for its members and patients.
National Abortion Federation (NAF)	A standards-based membership organization of abortion facilities (clinics, physicians' offices, and hospitals). To qualify for and maintain NAF membership, providers must meet NAF clinical and safety standards. The standards are revised annually to reflect current evidence and are the basis for members' certification.
Royal College of Obstetricians and Gynaecologists (RCOG)	A global reproductive health professional society based in the United Kingdom. Its more than 14,000 members include individuals involved in obstetrics or gynecology worldwide. RCOG's mission is to improve the standard of care and to advance the science and practice of obstetrics and gynecology.
Society of Family Planning (SFP)	A professional membership organization for qualified individuals who have an interest in family planning demonstrated through training, clinical or laboratory practice, or academic publication. SFP develops clinical guidelines and supports research on contraception and abortion.
World Health Organization (WHO)	The international public health organization of the United Nations, based in Geneva, Switzerland. WHO develops clinical guidelines on reproductive health care with the stated objective of improving health outcomes.

SOURCES: ACOG, 2017a; NAF, 2017b; RCOG, 2017; SFP, 2017; WHO, 2017.

be provided evidence-based information on their procedure options so they can make an informed and independent decision.

There is little evidence on how preabortion care is typically provided, but there is consensus among professional guidelines that the preabortion encounter includes the following elements (Baker and Beresford, 2009; NAF, 2017a; RCOG, 2015; WHO, 2014):

- individualized, sensitive, and respectful communication;
- cultural sensitivity;
- review of the risks and benefits of the available abortion procedures that is based on evidence and is easy to understand;
- options for pain management, including nonpharmaceutical approaches, analgesia, sedation, and anesthesia;
- support for emotional and other needs as they arise;
- confirmation that the abortion decision is voluntary (not coerced);

- explanation of what will be done before, during, and after the procedure, including the preabortion evaluation;
- description of what the patient is likely to experience, clear instruction on aftercare, and how to recognize potential complications requiring emergency care;
- whom to call and where to go for services for both routine and follow-up care; and
- information and counseling on future prevention of unintended pregnancy and contraceptive options, including the option to obtain contraception immediately following the procedure.

Patient education, counseling, and informed consent are overlapping components of preabortion care. Patient education refers to the information women should receive regarding the available treatment options and the risks and benefits of these options (Baker and Beresford, 2009). It is also integral to the informed consent process—a legal and ethical obligation to all patients defined by state and federal law, malpractice standards, and professional standards (ACOG, 2015; AMA, 2016; Joint Commission Resources, 2016; Kinnersley et al., 2013). Counseling involves addressing the patient's emotions, expectations, and beliefs about abortion care (Baker and Beresford, 2009).

Health care providers are legally required to obtain patients' informed consent before performing a medical procedure. Specific definitions of informed consent may vary from state to state, but the goal of the informed consent process is well established: to ensure that patients understand the nature and risks of the procedure they are considering and that their decision to undergo it is voluntary (AAAHC, 2016; AMA, 2016; HHS, 2017a; Joint Commission, 2016). The discussion should also include options for analgesia, sedation, or anesthesia, including their associated risks and benefits (AANA, 2016; ASA Committee on Ethics, 2016).

Not every woman wants or needs psychological counseling in addition to patient education before an abortion (Baker and Beresford, 2009; Baron et al., 2015; Brown, 2013; Moore et al., 2011). Some women may wish to discuss the emotional aspects of the abortion with a counselor (Moore et al., 2011), and individualized counseling may be helpful for women having difficulty with their decision (Baker and Beresford, 2009). Women should also be referred to and have access to additional counseling and social services if needed (e.g., for counseling on intimate partner violence, sexual abuse care, rape crisis counseling, mental health services, substance abuse services, and postabortion counseling) (Goodman et al., 2016). As noted in Chapter 1, most women who undergo abortions are poor or low-income. Three-quarters of abortion patients have family incomes below 200 percent of the federal poverty level (Jerman et al., 2016) and thus may benefit from social support services. In addition, although the evidence is drawn largely from non-U.S. data (Australia, Canada, China, New Zealand, and the United Kingdom), epidemiological studies have shown that women who have abortions are disproportionately at risk of interpersonal and other types of violence (Bourassa and Berube, 2007; Evins and Chescheir, 1996; Fanslow et al., 2008; Fisher et al., 2005; Glander et al., 1998; Janssen et al., 2003; Keeling et al., 2004; Leung et al., 2002; Russo and Denious, 2001; Saftlas et al., 2010; Steinberg and Russo, 2008; Taft and Watson, 2007; Taft et al., 2004). Little is known about the extent to which abortion patients receive the follow-up social and psychological supports they need. A study of Finnish registry data provides some evidence that monitoring for mental health status in a follow-up visit after abortion may help reduce the consequences of serious mental health disorders (Gissler et al., 2015).

Providing evidence-based information on how to prevent a future unintended pregnancy—including the option to obtain contraception contemporaneously with the procedure—is a standard component of abortion care (Goodman et al., 2016; NAF, 2017a; RCOG, 2015; WHO, 2014). Contraception discussions should be patient-centered, based on principles of informed consent using evidence-based information on the contraceptive alternatives, and guided by the patient's preferences (Goodman et al., 2016; RCOG, 2015). Most contraceptive methods can be administered safely immediately after an abortion (Fox et al., 2011; Goodman et al., 2016; Grimes et al., 2010; Okusanya et al., 2014; Patil et al., 2016; Sääv et al., 2012; WHO, 2014). Recent studies suggest improved contraceptive use with the placement of implants or the initiation of other contraceptive methods at the time of the abortion or when mifepristone is administered for an early medication abortion (Hognert et al., 2016; Raymond et al., 2016a; Whaley and Burke, 2015).

While numerous options for contraception are available, long-acting reversible contraception (LARC) methods are the most effective for pregnancy prevention (ACOG, 2017b; Winner et al., 2012). Further, they are associated with higher rates of continuation, even for adolescents and young women, and fewer repeat abortions compared with other forms of contraception (ACOG, 2017b; Ames and Norman, 2012; Diedrich et al., 2015; Goodman et al., 2008; Goyal et al., 2017; Kilander et al., 2016; Rose and Lawton, 2012; Rosenstock et al., 2012; Winner et al., 2012). A prospective cohort study of women of reproductive age in the St. Louis area—the Contraceptive CHOICE project—assessed the impact of an educational intervention designed to increase awareness of LARC among women who wanted to avoid pregnancy for at least 1 year. The 10,000 women who enrolled in the project had the opportunity to obtain the contraceptive method of their choice at no cost in a variety of clinical settings where they received family planning, obstetrical, gynecological, and primary care (including two facilities providing abortion care) (McNicholas et al., 2014; Secura et al., 2010). The study found that offering LARC at the time of enrollment was well received; 75 percent of the 9,256 participants opted for intrauterine devices (IUDs) or implants. LARC users were more likely than non-LARC users to continue using contraception at 12 and 24 months (86 percent versus 55 percent at 12 months, 77 percent versus 41 percent at 24 months). The generalizability of these findings, however, is uncertain given that the contraceptives were free, and the study population included only women who wanted to avoid pregnancy. The CHOICE study also evaluated a structured approach to contraceptive counseling and found that counseling could be provided effectively by trained personnel without a medical background (Madden et al., 2013).

INITIAL CLINICAL ASSESSMENT

Abortion care should always begin with a clinical evaluation, including a pertinent medical history and clinical assessment to assess the presence of comorbidities or contraindications relevant to the procedure. The primary aim of the evaluation is to confirm an intrauterine pregnancy and determine gestation. The physical exam may involve laboratory tests and ultrasonography to confirm an intrauterine pregnancy; assess gestation; screen for sexually transmitted infections (STIs) and cervical infections; document Rh status; or evaluate uterine size, position, and possible anomalies (ACOG and SFP, 2014; Goldstein and Reeves, 2009; Goodman et al., 2016; NAF, 2017a; RCOG, 2015; WHO, 2014). Women whose Rh status is unknown should be offered Rh testing and, if Rh negative, offered Rh immune globulin (ACOG and SFP, 2014, NAF, 2017a; RCOG, 2015). No evidence, however, indicates that Rh immune globulin is needed in pregnancies under 8 weeks' gestation (NAF, 2017a). While it should not delay the abortion procedure, screening for STIs may be appropriate if available (NAF, 2017a; RCOG, 2015). The contraindications and other circumstances affecting the appropriateness of each abortion method are discussed later in the chapter.

Pregnancy is dated from the first day of the last menstrual period (LMP) and is commonly measured by days' or weeks' gestation (Goldstein and Reeves, 2009). Either clinical evaluation or ultrasound examination can be used to establish gestation (ACOG and SFP, 2014; WHO, 2014). Ultrasound is not required, however, and there is no direct evidence that it improves the safety or effectiveness of the abortion (Kaneshiro et al., 2011; NAF, 2017a; Raymond et al., 2015; RCOG, 2015). In a study of nearly 4,500 medication abortion patients aimed at assessing the feasibility and efficacy of foregoing routine use of ultrasound, Bracken and colleagues (2011) found that LMP date combined with physical examination was highly effective at determining eligibility for medication abortion—patients accurately assessed their eligibility (Bracken et al., 2011).

SAFETY AND EFFECTIVENESS OF CURRENT ABORTION METHODS

Several methods—medication, aspiration, dilation and evacuation (D&E), and induction—are used to perform an abortion depending on weeks' gestation, patient preference, provider skill, need and desire for sedation, costs, clinical setting, and state policies and regulations.

Medication Abortion

Medication abortion in early pregnancy is accomplished using mifepristone, a progesterone receptor antagonist that competitively interacts with progesterone at the progesterone receptor site, thereby inhibiting the activity of endogenous or exogenous progesterone. This process initiates the breakdown of the endometrium and implanted embryo (Borkowski et al., 2015). Mifepristone, sold under the brand name Mifeprex,[1] is the only medication specifically approved by the FDA for use in medication abortion (Woodcock, 2016). Taken orally, it has been shown to increase sensitivity to prostaglandins and is most commonly used in conjunction with misoprostol, a prostaglandin E1 analogue. Misoprostol causes uterine contractions as well as cervical ripening and can be administered orally, sublingually, buccally, or vaginally.[2] Since mifepristone's initial FDA approval in 2000, an extensive body of research has led to improvements in the drug's protocol, including a lower recommended dosage, an increased period of eligibility from 49 days' to 70 days' (10 weeks') gestation, and a recommendation that the misoprostol be taken buccally rather than sublingually or orally to minimize side effects (Borkowski et al., 2015; Chai et al., 2013). The World Health Organization (WHO) has included mifepristone and misoprostol on its Model List of Essential Medicines since 2005 (WHO, 2015).[3]

Few women have contraindications to medication abortion (ACOG and SFP, 2014). The FDA-approved Mifeprex label states that the drug should not be used for women with confirmed or suspected ectopic pregnancy or undiagnosed adnexal mass; an IUD in place; chronic adrenal

---

[1]Mifeprex is manufactured and distributed by Danco Laboratories. Danco is the only distributer of Mifeprex in the United States.

[2]A sublingual medication is dissolved under the tongue. Buccal medications are placed between the gums and the cheek.

[3]Where permitted under national law and where culturally acceptable (WHO, 2015).

BOX 2-1
FDA Risk Evaluation and Mitigation Strategy (REMS)
Program for Mifeprex

The FDA REMS program restricts the chain of supply of certain drug products to ensure that the drugs are distributed only by authorized prescribers or pharmacies under specified conditions. The FDA considers the following when determining the necessity of a REMS:

- estimated size of the population likely to use the drug involved;
- seriousness of the disease or condition that is to be treated with the drug;
- expected benefit of the drug with respect to such disease or condition;
- expected or actual duration of treatment with the drug;
- seriousness of any known or potential adverse events that may be related to the drug and the background incidence of such events in the population likely to use the drug; and
- whether the drug is a new molecular entity.

As of March 2017, there were 77 approved REMS programs, including that of Mifeprex. A drug requiring a REMS must have at least one of the following:

- a Medication Guide for consumers;
- a communication plan for health care providers; and
- one of six "elements to assure safe use" of the medication (e.g., specifications for prescribers, places and conditions where the drug can be dispensed, and patient monitoring).

The FDA first established a REMS program for Mifeprex in 2011 and revised it in March 2016 along with an update to the drug's label. The revised

---

failure; concurrent long-term systemic corticosteroid therapy; hemorrhagic disorders or concurrent anticoagulant therapy; allergy to mifepristone, misoprostol, or other prostaglandins; or inherited porphyrias (FDA, 2016a).

Since 2011, the distribution and use of Mifeprex has been restricted under the requirements of the FDA Risk Evaluation and Mitigation Strategy (REMS) program (see Box 2-1). (See Chapter 3 for additional details on REMS requirements for clinicians who prescribe Mifeprex.) Despite the restriction, use of the medication method is increasing, especially in early pregnancy. As noted in Chapter 1, the percentage of all abortions by medication rose by 110 percent between 2004 and 2013 and is expected to increase further (Jatlaoui et al., 2016). In 2014, medication abortions accounted for approximately 45 percent of all U.S. abortions performed <9 weeks' gestation (Jones and Jerman, 2017).

REMS requirements do not differ substantially from the original. They include the following:

- Mifeprex may be dispensed only to patients in clinics, hospitals, or medical offices under the supervision of a certified prescriber. It cannot be dispensed through retail pharmacies.
- To be certified, health care providers must submit a Prescriber Agreement to the drug's distributor, Danco Laboratories, attesting to their ability to assess duration of pregnancy and to diagnose ectopic pregnancy. They must be able to provide or arrange for surgical intervention as well as access to medical facilities equipped to provide blood transfusions and resuscitation, if necessary. Nonphysicians, such as certified nurse-midwives and other advanced practice clinicians, may prescribe Mifeprex if they have prescription authority under state law.
- Before patients receive the drug, the prescriber must provide the patient the FDA-approved Medication Guide, fully explain the potential risks related to the treatment regimen, and review and complete the Patient Agreement form with the patient.

The revised label

- lowered the recommended Mifeprex dosage to 200 mg;
- extended the gestation period appropriate for its use from 49 days' to 70 days' (10 weeks') gestation;
- eliminated the requirement for an in-person follow-up visit; and
- eliminated mandatory reporting of nonfatal adverse events.

SOURCES: Borkowski et al., 2015; Dabrowska, 2017; FDA, 2016a,b,c; Gassman et al., 2017; Woodcock, 2016.

Effectiveness of the Current Medication Regimen

The current FDA-approved regimen for medication abortion is 200 mg of mifepristone taken orally, followed by 800 mcg of misoprostol taken buccally 24 to 48 hours later (FDA, 2016a). A recent systematic review of this regimen—including 33,846 medication abortions—found an overall effectiveness rate of 96.7 percent for gestations up to 63 days (9 weeks) (Chen and Creinin, 2015).[4]

---

[4]The review also included 332 abortions that were performed between 64 and 70 days' gestation; the efficacy rate for these procedures was 93.1 percent.

Reversal of Medication Abortion

There has recently been media attention to claims that medication abortions can be "reversed" by taking progesterone after the mifepristone but before taking the misoprostol (Graham, 2017). The claims are based on a case series report of seven patients who did not receive standardized doses or formulations of the medications (i.e., mifepristone or progesterone) (Delgado and Davenport, 2012). Case series are descriptive reports that are considered very low-quality evidence for drawing conclusions about a treatment's effects (Guyatt et al., 2011). In a related subsequent systematic review, Grossman and colleagues (2015) assessed the likelihood of a pregnancy continuing if the abortion medication regimen is not completed (i.e., the mifepristone dosage is not followed by misoprostol). However, the review found that there were insufficient data to conclude that the progesterone treatment is more likely to lead to continued pregnancy compared with expectant management after mifepristone alone.

Expected Side Effects

It is common for medical procedures to result in side effects in addition to the intended outcome. Medication abortions involve cramping, pain, and bleeding, similar to the symptoms of a miscarriage (ACOG and SFP, 2014; Borkowski et al., 2015; FDA, 2016a). Vaginal bleeding is expected during and after an abortion and occurs in almost all patients during a medication abortion (FDA, 2016a). Bleeding generally starts as the tissue begins to separate from the endometrium and continues for several days after the abortion is complete. The heaviest bleeding occurs during and immediately following the passage of the gestational sac and lasts 1 to 2 days. Some bleeding and spotting may occur up to 9–16 days.

Like bleeding, uterine pain and cramping are an expected and normal consequence of medication abortion (FDA, 2016a). Cramping can last from a half-day to 3 days (Ngo et al., 2011). Nonsteroidal anti-inflammatory drugs (NSAIDs) are typically recommended to manage the pain. Ibuprofen—after the onset of cramping—has been shown to reduce both pain and later analgesia use (Jackson and Kapp, 2011; Livshits et al., 2009). However, some women still report high levels of pain, and pain is commonly reported as the worst feature of the method. Prophylactic regimens for pain management are an area of active research (Dragoman et al., 2016).

Other side effects reported by women who undergo medication abortion include nausea, vomiting, weakness, diarrhea, headache, dizziness, fever, and chills (Chen and Creinin, 2015; FDA, 2016a). About 85 percent of patients report at least one of these side effects, and many patients are expected to report more than one (FDA, 2016a).

Complications

Complications after medication abortion, such as hemorrhage, hospitalization, persistent pain, infection, or prolonged heavy bleeding, are rare—occurring in no more than a fraction of a percent of patients (Chen and Creinin, 2015; FDA, 2016a; Ireland et al., 2015; Kulier et al., 2011; Woodcock, 2016). Obesity (i.e., a body mass index [BMI] of 30 or greater) has not been found to increase the risk for adverse outcomes after medication abortion (Strafford et al., 2009). The Society of Family Planning suggests that medication abortion may be preferable to aspiration abortion when patients, including those with extreme obesity, are at risk of procedural and anesthetic complications (SFP, 2012).

Hemorrhage   Prolonged heavy bleeding is rare but may indicate an incomplete abortion[5] or other complications. Hemorrhage requiring assessment or treatment following medication abortion is also rare. The FDA advises that women contact a health care provider immediately if bleeding after a medication abortion soaks through two thick full-size sanitary pads per hour for two consecutive hours (FDA, 2016a). In a study of 11,319 medication abortions performed in California between 2009 and 2010, hemorrhage occurred in 16 cases (0.14 percent) (Upadhyay et al., 2015).

The need for a blood transfusion—an uncommon occurrence—is an indication of clinically significant hemorrhage. In a study of more than 1,000 women receiving medication abortion in Norway, 1 patient required a transfusion (0.1 percent) and 32 required an aspiration procedure because of continued bleeding (3.0 percent) (Løkeland et al., 2014). In Chen and Creinin's (2015) systematic review of 20 studies and 33,846 women (described above), 0.03 to 0.6 percent of women required a blood transfusion after a medication abortion.

Infection   Serious infection occurs rarely after medication abortion; reports of fatal sepsis are exceedingly rare (<1 in 100,000) (FDA, 2011; Woodcock, 2016). Signs and symptoms of serious infection are fever of 100.4°F or higher lasting more than 4 hours, tachycardia, severe abdominal pain, pelvic tenderness, or general malaise with or without fever occurring more than 24 hours after administration of misoprostol (ACOG and SFP, 2014; FDA, 2016a). There is no evidence of a causal relationship between use of mifepristone and misoprostol and an increased risk of infection or death (FDA, 2016a; Woodcock, 2016). The incidence of infection in recent studies ranges from 0.01 to 0.5 percent (Chen and Creinin, 2015; Cleland et

---

[5]An "incomplete abortion" occurs when parts of the products of conception are retained in the uterus.

al., 2013; Upadhyay et al., 2015). According to the FDA's Adverse Event Reporting System, there were nine reports of severe bacterial infections following medication abortion from November 1, 2012, through April 30, 2015 (Woodcock, 2016). The FDA has concluded that the available evidence does not support the use of prophylactic antibiotics for medication abortion (CDER, 2016).

Need for uterine aspiration   Some women require a uterine aspiration after medication abortion because of retained products of conception, persistent pain or bleeding, or ongoing pregnancy (Chen and Creinin, 2015; Cleland et al., 2013; Ireland et al., 2015; Raymond et al., 2013; Upadhyay et al., 2015). Ireland and colleagues (2015) analyzed more than 13,000 electronic medical records documenting the outcomes of medication abortions (up to 9 weeks' gestation) performed in private Los Angeles clinics from November 2010 to August 2013. Of these, 2.1 percent required an unanticipated uterine aspiration either because of an ongoing pregnancy (0.4 percent) or for persistent pain, bleeding, or both (1.8 percent). Other recent estimates of the need for an unanticipated uterine aspiration range from 1.8 to 4.2 percent (Chen and Creinin, 2015). Rates vary in part because of differences in study populations (including weeks' gestation) and in treatment regimens (Cleland et al., 2013; Raymond et al., 2013; Upadhyay et al., 2015).

Impact of Clinical Setting on the Safety and Effectiveness of Medication Abortion

There is no direct evidence suggesting that specific types of facilities (e.g., ambulatory surgery centers or hospitals) or facility factors (e.g., size of procedure room or corridor width) are needed to ensure the safety of medication abortion. Indeed, most women in the United States return home after taking mifepristone and take the misoprostol 28 to 48 hours later. As a result, medication abortions occur largely in nonclinical settings. Moreover, as described above, a body of research including systematic reviews (Chen and Creinin, 2015; Kulier et al., 2011; Raymond et al., 2013) and large cohort studies (Cleland et al., 2013; Ireland et al., 2015; Upadhyay et al., 2015) demonstrates that complications such as infection, hemorrhage requiring transfusion, or hospitalization occur in fewer than 1.0 percent of patients.

Some research has focused specifically on medication abortion outside the hospital or clinic setting. A variety of studies, for example, have assessed the self-administration of misoprostol after receiving mifepristone in a clinic. This largely observational research shows that home use of misoprostol produces outcomes similar to those of the clinic-supervised method (Clark et al., 2005; Fiala et al., 2004; Guengant et al., 1999; Løkeland et al., 2014; Ngoc et al., 2004; Shannon et al., 2005; Shrestha and Sedhai, 2014).

Other research has assessed the safety and effectiveness of home use of both mifepristone and misoprostol (Chong et al., 2015; Conkling et al., 2015; Platais et al., 2016). In one U.S. prospective nonrandomized study, 400 women with pregnancies up to 63 days' gestation were offered the choice of either clinic-supervised or home use of mifepristone. Of these women, 128 chose home administration, and 272 chose clinic administration; the women did not differ significantly in terms of gravidity, gestation, or other measured characteristics. The women choosing home use were slightly older (27.8 versus 26.0 years) and more likely to be doing paid work (78.9 versus 68.0 percent). Success rates did not differ between the groups (96.3 versus 96.9 percent), and the 2 patients who required hospitalization were in the clinic-supervised group. One patient was diagnosed with an incomplete abortion and underwent a follow-up dilation and curettage procedure, and the other was treated for severe nausea and vomiting (Chong et al., 2015). A related study found that among 301 women offered the choice of home use, the factor most cited by women who chose this option was flexibility in scheduling (Swica et al., 2013).

Telemedicine

Telemedicine is the use of telecommunications and information technology to provide access to health assessment, diagnosis, intervention, consultation, supervision, and information across distance (HHS, 2017b). For medication abortion, the process involves a health care provider's reviewing the relevant medical information and having a discussion with the patient via teleconference. If clinical criteria are met, the health care provider remotely dispenses or issues a prescription for the medication abortion regimen (Aiken et al., 2018; Grossman et al., 2011a). Grossman and colleagues (2011a) investigated the effectiveness and acceptability of telemedicine for medication abortion (mean days' gestation was 47 days) compared with face-to-face physician visits in Iowa. Roughly half of the 578 patients were enrolled in the telemedicine option. The success rates for the two options were similar: 98.7 percent for the telemedicine patients and 96.9 percent for the clinic patients. No patient in either group required hospitalization, and there was no significant difference in the occurrence of adverse events. One of the 223 patients in the telemedicine group received a blood transfusion. In a recent 7-year retrospective cohort study in Iowa, researchers compared the rate of clinically significant adverse events (hospital admission, surgery, blood transfusion, emergency department treatment, or death) after medication abortion for 8,765 telemedicine patients and 10,405 in-person patients (Grossman and Grindlay, 2017). The overall rate of adverse events was less than 0.3 percent. The difference between the telemedicine patients (0.18 percent) and in-person patients (0.32 percent) was not statistically significant and was within the authors' margin of noninferiority. This finding indicates that telemedicine provision of medication abortion was not associated with a significantly higher prevalence of adverse events compared with in-person provision.

These reported risks are both low and similar in magnitude to the reported risks of serious adverse effects of commonly used prescription and over-the-counter medications. For example, it has been estimated that the use of NSAIDs is responsible for 3,500 hospitalizations and 400 deaths per year in UK residents aged 60 or older, a risk rate of 0.23 and 0.03 percent, respectively (Hawkey and Langman, 2003). The NSAID-related risk of hospitalization in elderly Medicaid patients in the United States has been estimated to be even higher—1.25 percent in one study (Smalley et al., 1995). The risk of diarrhea with many common antibiotics is as high as 39 percent (McFarland, 1998), and the risk of hospitalization due to the more serious *Clostridium difficile* infection may be as high as 0.02 percent with some antibiotic combinations (Hirschhorn et al., 1994). Taken together, these findings provide additional indirect evidence that no facility-specific factors are needed to ensure the safety of medication abortion, as there is no perceived need for facility-specific factors to ensure the safety of these other common pharmaceuticals. These safety data accord with professional guidelines or best practices according to which routine early medication abortion does not require sophisticated settings and can be safely performed in settings typical for the delivery of women's health care and family planning services (ACOG and SFP, 2014; NAF, 2017a; RCOG, 2015; WHO, 2014).

In their analysis of the Iowa study described above, Grossman and colleagues (2013) conducted a geographic analysis to assess the effect of the telemedicine model on access to medication abortion for women in different areas of the state. They found that the proportion of all Iowa abortions that were medication abortions had increased, from 33.4 to 45.3 percent (p <.001), in the 2-year periods before and after telemedicine was introduced. The increase was especially notable among women living in more remote areas. Women who lived more than 50 miles from an abortion clinic that provided only surgical abortions were 16 percent more likely to have a medication abortion (adjusted odds ratio [aOR] = 1.16; 95% confidence interval [CI] = 1.05, 1.28). The proportion of medication abortions at the study sites had also increased from 46 to 54 percent after telemedicine was introduced (p <.001). Overall, women in Iowa had a 46 percent greater likelihood of having an earlier abortion (<14 weeks' gestation) (aOR = 1.46; 95% CI = 1.22, 1.75).

Aspiration Abortion

Aspiration is a minimally invasive and commonly used gynecological procedure (Meckstroth and Paul, 2009; Roblin, 2014).[6] The procedure time is typically less than 10 minutes (Edelman et al., 2001; Goldberg et al., 2004). As noted in the previous chapter, aspiration is currently the most common abortion method used in the United States regardless of gestation, accounting for almost 68 percent of abortions in 2013.[7] The method may be used up to 14 to 16 weeks' gestation. Aspiration is also used in cases of early pregnancy loss (miscarriage) and management of incomplete abortion for medication abortion.

The first steps in the procedure are cervical dilation and priming (when appropriate) so that the contents of the uterus can be evacuated. Cervical dilation is usually done using tapered mechanical dilators and is recommended over routine priming except for adolescents and others for whom cervical dilation may be challenging (Allen and Goldberg, 2016). Cervical priming is accomplished with either osmotic dilators[8] or pharmacological agents (e.g., misoprostol), or both. When placed in the cervix, the osmotic dilator absorbs moisture from the tissues surrounding the cervix and gradually swells to slowly open the cervical orifice (os). The pharmaceutical agents are prostaglandin analogues or progesterone antagonists, such as the drug misoprostol, which is also used in medication abortion.

After cervical dilation and, when indicated, priming, a suction cannula (plastic or metal tube) is inserted through the cervix into the uterus. The cannula is attached to a vacuum source—an electric vacuum pump for electric vacuum aspiration or a handheld, hand-activated aspirator (syringe) for manual vacuum aspiration—to empty the uterine contents. Ultrasound guidance is sometimes used (RCOG, 2011).

See later in this chapter for a discussion of the use of sedation and anesthesia during abortion procedures, including the implications for personnel needs and facility requirements.

---

[6]There is no standard terminology for this type of abortion. As noted in Chapter 1, this report uses the term "aspiration abortion," although others commonly refer to the same procedure as "surgical abortion," "vacuum aspiration," "suction curettage," or "suction evacuation."

[7]Centers for Disease Control and Prevention (CDC) surveillance reports use the catchall category of "curettage" to refer to nonmedical abortion methods. The committee assumed that CDC curettage estimates before 13 weeks' gestation refer to aspiration procedures and that curettage estimates after 13 weeks' gestation are D&E procedures.

[8]Laminaria, small tubes made of dried seaweed, and manmade sterile sponges are common types of osmotic dilators.

Effectiveness of Aspiration Abortion

Recent comparisons of aspiration and medication abortion methods indicate that aspiration may be only slightly more effective than medication abortion in early pregnancy. In Ireland and colleagues' (2015) study of private Los Angeles clinics described in the prior section, the efficacy rate for almost 17,000 aspiration abortions performed up to 9 weeks' gestation was 99.8 percent, compared with 99.6 percent for medication abortions[9] for the same gestational period (Ireland et al., 2015).

Expected Side Effects

As in medication abortion, bleeding, uterine pain, and cramping are expected and normal consequences of aspiration abortion.

Complications

Aspiration abortions rarely result in complications. In a recent retrospective analysis of California fee-for-service Medicaid claims data, 57 of almost 35,000 women (0.16 percent) were found to have experienced a serious complication (hospital admission, surgery, or blood transfusion) after an aspiration abortion (Upadhyay et al., 2015). A systematic review on aspiration-related complications documents a somewhat higher complication rate (ranging from 0 to 5 percent), but a large proportion of the studies in that review included now outdated procedures, including dilation and sharp curettage (White et al., 2015).

In a historical cohort study, Guiahi and colleagues (2015) analyzed the outpatient medical records of women who had undergone an aspiration abortion between January 2009 and March 2014 in a Colorado clinic. The researchers compared the outcomes of women with (n = 587) and without (n = 1,373) medical comorbidities, including diabetes, hypertension, obesity (weight ≥200 lb or BMI ≥30), HIV, epilepsy, asthma, thyroid disease, and/or bleeding and clotting disorders having aspiration abortions. The researchers found no difference in the rate of complications between the women with at least one comorbidity and those with no comorbidity (odds ratio [OR] = 0.9; 95% CI = 0.5, 1.6).

Need for repeat aspiration   Repeat aspiration is most often required for retained products of conception after an abortion. Rates of <0.1 to 8.0 percent have been reported for this complication, related to gestation, experience of the provider, and use of ultrasound guidance (White et al., 2015).

---

[9]$p < .001$.

Studies showing the highest rates of repeat aspiration included women at ≤6 weeks' gestation and were conducted more than 20 years ago (Bassi et al., 1994). Tissue inspection is recommended after aspiration abortion, regardless of gestation, but products of conception may be difficult to identify prior to 7 weeks' gestation (NAF, 2017a; SFP, 2013). Additional protocols, including magnification of aspirate, follow-up by serum beta-hCG estimation, and flotation of tissue with backlighting may be used to confirm abortion completion (NAF, 2017a; RCOG, 2011; SFP, 2013).

Hemorrhage   Hemorrhage requiring transfusion or other treatment (medication administration or repeat aspiration) complicates 0.0 to 4.7 percent of aspiration abortions, with more recent studies reporting a rate of 1.3 percent (Upadhyay et al., 2015; White et al., 2015). In the California Medicaid study, 0.13 percent of aspiration procedures were complicated by hemorrhage (Upadhyay et al., 2015).

Infection   Current clinical guidelines recommend routine antibiotic prophylaxis before all aspiration abortions (NAF, 2017a; RCOG, 2015; SFP, 2011b; WHO, 2014). Like any invasive procedure, aspiration abortion carries some risk of infection. If untreated, an upper genital tract infection subsequent to abortion can lead to chronic pelvic pain, dyspareunia, ectopic pregnancy, and infertility (Low et al., 2012). Serious infection after aspiration, however, is rare. In a 2012 systematic review, the Cochrane Collaboration evaluated the effectiveness of perioperative antibiotics in preventing upper genital tract infection (including infection of the uterus and fallopian tubes) (Low et al., 2012). The researchers concluded that universal antibiotic prophylaxis is effective in preventing infection after an aspiration procedure: the incidence of upper genital tract infection among women who received prophylactic antibiotics was 59 percent of that among women who received a placebo. The rate of infection was 5.8 percent among women who received antibiotics (n = 3,525) and 9.4 percent among women in the placebo group (n = 3,500).

In a more recent systematic review of complications following aspiration abortion (up to 14 weeks' gestation), White and colleagues (2015) report that 0.0 to 0.4 percent of 188,395 women undergoing aspiration abortions required intravenous (IV) antibiotics after the procedure in 11 of 12 office-based settings. In Upadhyay and colleagues' (2015) analysis of almost 35,000 aspiration abortions in California, 94 women (0.27 percent) developed an infection after the procedure. Most infections after outpatient aspiration procedures are treated with oral antibiotics, with up to 0.4 percent of patients with infection requiring IV antibiotic administration (White et al., 2015).

Uterine perforation   Uterine perforation involves injury to the uterine wall, as well as potential injury to other abdominal organs. While the risk of uterine perforation in older studies has been reported as ≤0.1 to 2.3 percent, the majority of more recent studies of aspiration abortion report no cases of uterine perforation or note that perforations that occurred were successfully managed conservatively without the need for additional surgery or hospitalization (White et al., 2015). In the study of almost 35,000 California Medicaid-covered aspiration abortions referenced above, 0.01 percent resulted in a perforation (Upadhyay et al., 2015).

Cervical laceration   Cervical laceration (injury to the cervix from instrumentation) is also very rare, with most studies reporting none or 1 case (<0.1 to 0.6 percent) (Ohannessian et al., 2016; White et al., 2015). In a study evaluating the risks of aspiration abortion in teens versus adults, an increased risk of cervical laceration was noted for adolescent patients (0.5 versus 0.2 percent), but this study was conducted prior to current approaches to cervical preparation (Cates et al., 1983; White et al., 2015). Use of osmotic dilators was common in older studies, but the more common approach today is medical, using misoprostol 2 to 3 hours prior to the procedure (Allen and Goldberg, 2016; O'Connell et al., 2009). While current recommendations do not include routine use of medical or mechanical cervical preparation because of the delay that would result, misoprostol is commonly used in nulliparous women and young adolescents between 12 and 14 weeks' gestation (Allen and Goldberg, 2016).

Dilation and Evacuation

Fewer than 9 percent of abortions in the United States occur after 13 weeks' gestation (Jatlaoui et al., 2016). The D&E method, sometimes referred to as a second-trimester surgical abortion, appears to account for the majority of procedures performed between 14 and 20 weeks' gestation. Precise estimates of the rate of abortions by type during these weeks are not available. Reports often cite CDC surveillance statistics as suggesting that D&Es account for up to 96 percent of abortions between 14 and 20 weeks' gestation (ACOG, 2013; Hammond and Chasen, 2009). However, the oft-cited CDC data are actually aggregate estimates that include not only D&E but also other methods (Jatlaoui et al., 2016; Pazol et al., 2009).

D&E techniques have evolved in the decades since the method was first developed (ACOG, 2013; Hammond and Chasen, 2009; Lohr et al., 2008). The procedure is typically performed in two stages, although the specific approaches to cervical preparation, instrumentation, and other aspects may vary (Grossman et al., 2008; Ibis Reproductive Health, 2015; Lohr et al., 2008). The procedure itself generally takes less than 30 minutes

(Ben-Ami et al., 2009; Grossman et al., 2008, 2011b). The first step is cervical preparation, dilating the cervix with laminaria (or other type of osmotic dilator) and/or a prostaglandin (e.g., misoprostol). Slow dilation is recommended (e.g., over a few hours, overnight, or sometime repeated over 24 to 48 hours) to minimize the need for supplemental manual or mechanical dilation (Grossman et al., 2008; Lohr et al., 2008). With a greater degree of dilation, the uterus is more easily emptied, instruments are easier to use, and procedure time is shortened (Hern, 2016). Once dilation is adequate and analgesia, sedation, and/or anesthesia have been administered, the amniotic fluid is aspirated (Lohr et al., 2008; WHO, 2014). Before 16 weeks' gestation, suction aspiration may suffice to empty the uterus. At 16 weeks, forceps extraction may also be required. Beyond 16 weeks, suction is not effective, and forceps should be used to remove fetal parts and the placenta. A curette and/or additional suction are also used to remove any remaining tissue or blood clots. Following the procedure, the provider examines the tissue to confirm that the evacuation was complete. Patients should be observed following the procedure to monitor for any postoperative complications (Hammond and Chasen, 2009; Lohr et al., 2008).

Ultrasonography is recommended so the physician can visualize the surgical instruments, locate fetal parts, and confirm an empty uterus (NAF, 2017a). Routine intraoperative ultrasonography has been demonstrated to significantly reduce the risk of uterine perforation and shorten the time required to complete the procedure (Darney and Sweet, 1989).

Performing D&E procedures requires advanced training and/or experience (Cates et al., 1982; Hern, 2016; Lohr et al., 2008; RCOG, 2015; WHO, 2012). Chapter 3 reviews the required clinical skills for performing abortions.

Complications

Although the risk of complications increases with weeks' gestation (Bartlett et al., 2004; Grossman et al., 2008; Zane et al., 2015), a range of retrospective cohort studies, case series, chart reviews, and a prospective case series have shown D&E to be effective with minimal rates of complications, ranging from 0.05 to 4 percent (ACOG, 2013; Autry et al., 2002; Bryant et al., 2011; Cates et al., 1982; Frick et al., 2010; Grimes et al., 1977; Grossman et al., 2008; Jacot et al., 1993; Mauelshagen et al., 2009; Peterson et al., 1983).

One study, however, suggests that a history of multiple prior cesarean deliveries may significantly increase the risk of a major complication. In a multivariable logistic analysis of 2,973 D&Es performed between 2004 and 2007 at an urban public hospital, Frick and colleagues (2010) found an overall rate of major complications (i.e., transfusion required; disseminated intravascular coagulation; or a reoperation involving uterine artery embolization, laparoscopy, or laparotomy) of about 1.0 percent. However, women with two or more prior cesarean sections had a sevenfold increased risk of a major complication (OR = 7.37; 95% CI = 3.35, 15.80) (Frick et al., 2010). A history of one prior cesarean section was not associated with an increased risk of complications, although the authors note that a larger sample might lead to different results.

Obesity has also been studied as a possible risk factor for women undergoing D&E abortions (Benson et al., 2016; Lederle et al., 2015; Murphy et al., 2012). In a retrospective cohort study of 4,968 women undergoing aspiration and D&E abortions at a large outpatient clinic in 2012–2014, obesity was not associated with increased risk of complications[10] (Benson et al., 2016). The same conclusion resulted from a retrospective cohort study of 4,520 D&Es performed in a hospital-based abortion practice in 2009–2013 and a retrospective review of 1,044 women undergoing D&E or dilation and suction (D&S)[11] between 13 and 24 weeks' gestation in 2007–2010 (Lederle et al., 2015; Murphy et al., 2012). Lederle and colleagues (2015) found no association between BMI and D&E complications[12] after adjustment for age, ethnicity, prior vaginal delivery, prior cesarean delivery, and gestational duration. Murphy and colleagues (2012) compared complication rates, operative times, and anesthesia times between obese and nonobese (BMI <30) women and found no significant difference in complication rates. Finally, a retrospective analysis of D&E procedures performed between 2009 and 2014 found an association between obesity and increased risk for complications[13] in abortions performed after 14 weeks' gestation (Mark et al., 2017). Complications increased by BMI category,[14] and the increase in

---

[10]Complications assessed included need for uterine reaspiration (including same-day reaspiration), uterine perforation, cervical laceration, infection, emergency department visit or hospitalization, and excessive blood loss (defined as estimated blood loss greater than or equal to 100 mL).

[11]Dilation and curettage/suction denoted procedures performed when no other instruments besides suction were used; 5.3 percent of procedures in the study were D&S.

[12]Complications assessed included cervical laceration, hemorrhage, uterine atony, anesthesia complications, uterine perforation, disseminated intravascular coagulation, retained products of conception, and major complications (defined as those requiring hospitalization, transfusion, or further surgical intervention).

[13]Complications assessed included hemorrhage, need for repeat evacuation, uterine perforation, cervical laceration, medication reaction, unexpected surgery, or unplanned admission to the hospital.

[14]The cohort was classified into categories based on the WHO classification of underweight (BMI <18.5), normal weight (BMI 18.5–24.9), overweight (BMI 25.0–29.9), obese Class I (BMI 30–34.9), obese Class II (BMI 35–39.9), and obese Class III (BMI 40 or greater).

complications in women with Class III obesity was significant (OR = 5.04; 95% CI = 1.65–15.39).

Hemorrhage In studies of abortions performed in the year 2000 or later, D&E-related hemorrhage requiring transfusion or other treatment occurred in 0.0 to 1.0 percent of cases (Frick et al., 2010; Grossman et al., 2011a; Mauelshagen et al., 2009).

Infection Routine antibiotic prophylaxis is recommended for all surgical abortions (ACOG, 2013; NAF, 2017a; RCOG, 2015; WHO, 2014). Infection after a D&E is uncommon, with rates ranging from 0.0 to 2.0 percent (Autry et al., 2002; Grossman et al., 2011a; Mauelshagen et al., 2009). In the California Medicaid study described above, Upadhyay and colleagues (2015) found that 0.3 percent or 18 of 8,837 abortions performed after 13 weeks' gestation resulted in an infection, although these procedures included both D&Es and inductions.

Cervical lacerations Injuries to the cervix and uterus have decreased significantly with routine cervical preparation prior to D&E (ACOG, 2013). Recent studies have reported rates of 0.02 to 3.3 percent (Autry et al., 2002; Frick et al., 2010). The risk of cervical laceration is associated with mechanical dilation, nulliparity, advanced gestation, and provider inexperience (ACOG, 2013). Thus, as noted above, performing D&E procedures requires advanced training and/or experience.

Uterine perforation While uterine perforation is more common in D&E than in aspiration procedures, the incidence remains quite low and is likely related to the availability of cervical preparation and ultrasound guidance (Grossman et al., 2008). Limited clinician experience and underestimation of the duration of pregnancy are also factors that have been associated with uterine perforation (Grossman et al., 2008). A 1989 study compared the incidence of perforation during 810 D&E procedures with and without sonography (Darney and Sweet, 1989). Using ultrasound to guide the use of intrauterine forceps clearly improved the safety of the procedure: the rate of perforation declined significantly from 1.4 to 0.2 percent. Studies dating from 2010 to 2015 report perforation rates ranging from 0.2 to 0.8 percent (Frick et al., 2010; Upadhyay et al., 2015).

The facility requirements that are appropriate for D&Es depend on the level of sedation and anesthesia that is used. (See later in this chapter for a review of the use of analgesia, sedation, and anesthesia during abortions.)

Induction Abortions

As noted in Chapter 1, abortion terminology can be confusing. All abortion methods are sometimes referred to as "induced," and the term "medical" is often used to describe any nonsurgical method regardless of how early or late in pregnancy it occurs. In this section, the term "induction abortion" refers specifically to nonsurgical abortions that use medications to induce labor and delivery of the fetus. Relevant research and clinical guidelines use varying lower and upper gestation limits. In practice, the gestational parameters for induction vary depending on the facility, patient and provider preference, and state laws and regulations (SFP, 2011a).

Induction abortions are rarely performed in the United States; in 2013, they accounted for approximately 2 percent of all abortions at 14 weeks' gestation or later (Jatlaoui et al., 2016). For many women in the United States, D&E is often the preferred alternative because induction is more painful, its timing is less predictable and slower (sometimes taking more than 24 hours), and it is more expensive (see below) (ACOG, 2013; Ashok et al., 2004; Grimes et al., 2004; Grossman et al., 2008; Kelly et al., 2010; Lohr et al., 2008). In some clinical settings, however, D&E is not an option because the available clinicians lack the necessary experience and/or training in D&E procedures (SFP, 2011a).[15] In addition, D&E abortions are illegal in Mississippi and West Virginia.[16]

Optimal Medication Regimen for Induction Abortions

The medication regimens for performing an induction abortion have evolved and improved in response to a growing body of research—most notably with respect to the combined use of mifepristone and misoprostol (Gemzell-Danielsson and Lalitkumar, 2008; Wildschut et al., 2011). The safety and efficacy of different medications and medication regimens for inducing abortion has been assessed in RCTs, retrospective analyses, prospective observational studies, and systematic reviews (Ashok et al., 2002, 2004; Constant et al., 2016; Goh and Thong, 2006; Gouk et al., 1999; Hamoda et al., 2003; Kapp et al., 2007; Mauelshagen et al., 2009; Ngoc et al., 2011; Sonalkar et al., 2017; Wildschut et al., 2011).

In a systematic review of the effectiveness and side effects of different induction abortion medication regimens, the Cochrane Collaboration identified 36 RCTs that used various agents and methods of administration. The researchers concluded that a combination of mifepristone and misoprostol

---

[15]See Chapter 3 for a review of factors contributing to the dearth of trained providers.

[16]Both states allow exceptions in cases of life endangerment or severe physical health risk to the woman.

is the most effective approach and requires the shortest amount of time (Wildschut et al., 2011).

Guidelines developed by the American College of Obstetricians and Gynecologists (ACOG) and endorsed by the Society of Family Planning (SFP) and the Society of Maternal-Fetal Medicine recommend an alternative misoprostol regimen when mifepristone is not available (ACOG, 2013). Although effective, misoprostol-only regimens take longer (Wildschut et al., 2011) and as a result, are likely to be more costly to the patient with respect to time, discomfort, and out-of-pocket expense.

The National Abortion Federation (NAF) guidelines note that, when performed by trained clinicians, induction abortions can be provided in medical offices, clinics, or higher-level health care facilities (NAF, 2017a).

Complications

The expected side effects of induction abortions are similar to those described above for medication abortions at or before 10 weeks' gestation: cramping, pain, and bleeding, as well as nausea, vomiting, diarrhea, chills, and headache (Borgatta, 2011; Ngoc et al., 2011; Wildschut et al., 2011). The side effects are a result of the medications that are used for induction, the abortion process itself, or the medications used to manage pain (Borgatta, 2011).

The literature on complications resulting from induction abortions is limited by a variety of factors. The available research is a mix of study designs analyzing a variety of treatment protocols and patient populations that differ in important ways, including weeks' gestation, parity, fetal anomaly, and the pharmaceutical regimens and agents used to induce labor (Goyal, 2009; SFP, 2011a). All of these factors may affect patient outcomes. Moreover, while the research on the outcomes of medication and aspiration abortions draws on the outcomes of thousands of patients, the study samples for research on inductions are relatively small and thus have limited statistical power. Nevertheless, the available evidence consistently finds that induction abortion rarely leads to serious complications, although they occur more often than in D&E procedures (Bryant et al., 2011; Grossman, et al., 2008; Mauelshagen et al., 2009; SFP, 2011b).

In addition, among women with a prior cesarean delivery, the use of prostaglandins (particularly misoprostol) to induce labor during a normal vaginal delivery has been associated with an increased risk of uterine rupture—a potentially life-threatening condition (Lydon-Rochelle et al., 2001). Because methods to induce abortion are similar to those used to induce vaginal deliveries, research has assessed whether women with a prior cesarean are at similar risk of uterine rupture when undergoing an induction abortion. The evidence suggests that misoprostol-induced abortions are safe after a cesarean. Uterine rupture has been documented in fewer than

0.4 percent of induction abortions among women with a prior cesarean (Berghella et al., 2009; Goyal, 2009).

POSTABORTION CARE

Clinical guidelines suggest that, regardless of abortion method, routine in-person follow-up care is not necessary. However, clinicians may choose to offer an in-person follow-up visit to women 7–14 days after the procedure to confirm the absence of ongoing pregnancy and to assess recovery (NAF, 2017a; WHO, 2014). In the case of medication abortion, which usually occurs in a nonclinical setting, confirmation of termination of the pregnancy is the primary concern after the abortion. The FDA advises that follow-up is needed to confirm complete termination of pregnancy, but that termination can be confirmed by medical history, clinical examination, hCG testing, or ultrasound (FDA, 2016a). Similarly, NAF advises that confirmation can be established by any of these methods in an office, by telephone, or through electronic communication (NAF, 2017a).

Before a woman leaves a facility after an abortion procedure (or after she has taken the appropriate medication in the case of medication abortion), she should receive instructions on what to expect after the procedure, self-care, resuming intercourse, recognizing signs and symptoms of complications, and how and where to seek assistance if needed (NAF, 2017a; RCOG, 2015; WHO, 2014). Fertility goals and future pregnancy should be discussed, and if a woman opts for contraceptive counseling or a method of contraception, it should be provided before she leaves the facility (NAF, 2017a; RCOG, 2016; WHO, 2014). Other treatment (pain medication, medication for RhD-negative patients, emotional support) and referrals for other services (STI/HIV counseling and testing, abuse support services, psychological or social services, and services of other physician specialists) should also be provided before discharge, as needed (RCOG, 2016; WHO, 2014).

As with any other procedure, women who receive minimal, moderate, or deeper sedation should be monitored continuously during a recovery period until they have been evaluated and determined to be no longer at risk for hemodynamic instability or respiratory depression (NAF, 2017a). Prior to discharge, women must be ambulatory with stable blood pressure and pulse, bleeding and pain must be controlled, and these criteria must be documented (NAF, 2017a).

USE OF ANALGESIA, SEDATION, AND ANESTHESIA IN ABORTION CARE

Patient comfort not only is of critical interest to the patient but also affects the ability of the clinician to perform a procedure safely and effectively (Allen et al., 2013). People differ in their experience of and tolerance for pain. In their review of pain relief for obstetrical and gynecological procedures in outpatient settings, Allen and colleagues (2013) observed that anxiety, depression, and a woman's expectation of pain are strong predictors of her actual experience of pain during a procedure.

NAF recommends that providers involve women in the analgesia/sedation/anesthesia decision and that the choice be based on the individual patient's needs and an assessment of the risks and benefits (NAF, 2017a). The pain management approach that is best for women undergoing medication, aspiration, D&E, or induction abortions depends not only on which method is used but also on weeks' gestation, the patient's preferences for pain control, her comorbidities (if any), the availability of equipment and specialized personnel, provider preferences, cost, and facility licensure (Allen et al., 2012, 2013; NAF, 2017a; Nichols et al., 2009; RCOG, 2015). Results of a 2002 survey of NAF administrators and providers offer some insight into providers' preferred methods for pain control during aspiration abortions. Almost half (46 percent) of the 110 survey respondents preferred using local and/or oral medication, 33 percent preferred local plus IV sedation, and 21 percent preferred deep sedation or general anesthesia (O'Connell et al., 2009). The survey also elicited information regarding pain control for D&E and induction abortions. Most clinics that offered combined local and IV conscious sedation or general anesthesia used these methods for more than 80 percent of their patients (O'Connell et al., 2008).

The literature on the effectiveness of nonpharmacological approaches to reducing pain during abortion is inconclusive (Tschann et al., 2016). While a variety of methods have been assessed, including relaxation techniques (e.g., focused breathing, visualization, vocal coaching, and positive suggestion), hypnosis, aromatherapy, and abortion doulas, more definitive research is needed.

Pain Management During Aspiration, D&E, and Induction Abortions

The pharmaceutical options for pain management during an abortion range from oral analgesics (e.g., NSAIDs), to local anesthesia (typically a paracervical block), to minimal sedation/anxiolysis, to moderate sedation/analgesia, to deep sedation/analgesia, to general anesthesia (NAF, 2017a). Along this continuum, the physiological effects of sedation have increasing clinical implications and, depending on the depth of sedation, may require special equipment and personnel to ensure the patient's safety (see Tables 2-2 and 2-3). The greatest risk of using sedative agents is respiratory depression.

The American Society of Anesthesiologists (ASA) issues clinical standards for the safe use of pain medications and anesthesia in the types

TABLE 2-2 Levels and Effects of Analgesia, Sedation, and Anesthesia

Effect on	Minimal Sedation/ Anxiolysis[a]	Moderate Sedation/ Analgesia[b]	Deep Sedation/ Analgesia	General Anesthesia
Responsiveness	Normal response to verbal stimulation	Purposeful response to verbal or tactile stimulation	Purposeful response with repeated or painful stimulation	Unarousable by painful stimulus
Airway	Unaffected	No intervention required	Intervention may be required	Intervention often required
Spontaneous ventilation	Unaffected	Adequate	May be inadequate	Frequently inadequate
Cardiovascular function	Unaffected	Usually maintained	Usually maintained	May be impaired

[a]Minimal sedation includes local anesthesia, e.g., in the form of a paracervical block.
[b]Moderate sedation is sometimes described as "conscious sedation."
SOURCES: ASA, 2015; ASA Task Force, 2002.

of outpatient clinical settings where abortions are provided (ASA, 2013, 2014b, 2015). The standards use a physical health classification system—ASA I through ASA VI—to guide clinicians' decisions about anesthesia options. ASA I patients are healthy, and ASA II patients have mild systemic disease;[17] both are medically eligible for all options up to deep sedation in office-based settings. The vast majority of abortion patients—young women—are in these categories. Women with severe systemic disease (ASA III and IV) require further medical assessment and may be eligible for deep sedation (monitored anesthesia care [MAC]) or general anesthesia in an accredited ambulatory surgery center (ASC) or hospital. Table 2-2 shows the ASA levels of sedation and their effects on cognitive, respiratory, and cardiovascular function.

Safeguards for Managing Complications and Emergencies During an Abortion

The key safeguards—for abortions and all outpatient procedures—are whether the facility has the appropriate equipment, personnel, and

---

[17]ASA II patients (mild systemic disease) have no functional limitations and well-controlled disease, such as controlled hypertension or diabetes (without systemic effects), mild lung disease, or mild obesity (BMI between 30 and 40) (ASA, 2014a).

TABLE 2-3 Minimum Facility Requirements Related to Level of Sedation for Medication, Aspiration, and Dilation and Evacuation (D&E) Abortions

Abortion Method	Minimum Facility Requirements[a]			
	Equipment to Monitor Oxygen Saturation, Heart Rate, and Blood Pressure	Equipment to Monitor Ventilation (e.g., end-tidal carbon dioxide)[b]	Emergency Resuscitation Equipment	Emergency Transfer Plan
Medication	—	—	—	—
Aspiration with moderate sedation[a]	√	—	√	√
D&E				
Deep sedation, or monitored anesthesia care (MAC)	√	√	√	√
General anesthesia	√	√	√	√

NOTES: Checkmarks denote American Society of Anesthesiologists (ASA) minimal facility requirements as they relate to the level of sedation used in medication, aspiration, and D&E abortions.

[a]These requirements are for healthy patients or patients with mild systemic disease, i.e., ASA physical health status classifications ASA I and ASA II. Women with severe systemic disease (i.e., ASA III and IV) should be evaluated, and consideration should be given to using deep sedation (MAC) or general anesthesia in an accredited facility such as an ambulatory surgery center or hospital.

[b]End-tidal carbon dioxide monitoring refers to the noninvasive measurement of exhaled carbon dioxide.

SOURCES: Allen et al., 2013; ASA, 2013, 2014a,b, 2015; ASA Task Force, 2002.

emergency transfer plan to address any complications that might occur. While data on the use of specific pain management methods during an abortion are very limited, studies that report outcomes for patients after an abortion find that current pain management methods are safe when appropriate precautions are followed (Dean et al., 2011; Gokhale et al., 2016; Renner et al., 2012).

Facility Requirements

Table 2-3 shows the ASA minimal facility requirements as they relate to the level of sedation used in medication, aspiration, and D&E abortions. No special equipment or emergency arrangements are required for medication abortions. If moderate sedation is used during an aspiration abortion, the facility should have emergency resuscitation equipment and an emergency transfer plan, as well as equipment to monitor oxygen saturation, heart rate, and blood pressure. D&Es that involve deep sedation or general anesthesia should be provided in similarly equipped facilities that also have equipment to monitor ventilation (e.g., end-tidal carbon dioxide) (ASA Task Force, 2002).

New insights into the safe provision of sedation and anesthesia for abortions in outpatient settings are forthcoming. A unique research project, currently ongoing, is comparing the relative safety, cost, and complications of providing abortions in office-based settings and ASCs (ANSIRH, 2017; Roberts, 2017). The investigators are using a national private insurance claims database containing approximately 50 million patient records to compare adverse events, including anesthesia-related outcomes, in the two settings. The study's results were not available when the committee prepared this report. However, analyses of large-scale databases suggest that the risk of hospital admission after outpatient surgery (involving deep sedation) is rare for healthy patients undergoing procedures that last less than 120 minutes (Fleisher et al., 2007). As noted earlier, aspiration abortions typically take 10 minutes, and D&E procedures less than 30 minutes.

Personnel Requirements

The use of sedation and anesthesia also has important implications for personnel. If moderate sedation is used, it is essential to have a nurse or other qualified clinical staff—in addition to the person performing the abortion—available to monitor the patient (ASA Task Force, 2002; NAF, 2017a). Both deep sedation and general anesthesia require the expertise of an anesthesiologist or certified registered nurse anesthetist (CRNA) to ensure patient safety.

Evidence on Complications of Analgesia, Sedation, and Anesthesia During Abortions

This section reviews the available evidence on complications related to pain management during aspiration, D&E, and induction abortions. As noted above, NSAIDs reduce the discomfort of pain and cramping safely and effectively during a medication abortion.

Aspiration Pain Management

Paracervical blocks are used routinely to reduce the pain of cervical dilation during aspiration procedures (Allen et al., 2013; Nichols et al., 2009). Moderate and deep sedation are also options for aspiration abortion. The blocks are effective in decreasing pain related to cervical dilation and uterine aspiration, although administration of the block itself is painful (Allen et al., 2013; Renner et al., 2012), and some providers use other medications to reduce the pain of the injection (Allen et al., 2013). Because some women report experiencing moderate to significant procedural pain even with the block, researchers are trying to identify an optimal approach to pain management without sedation during aspiration (Allen et al., 2013; O'Connell et al., 2009; Renner et al., 2012, 2016).

Adverse events related to the use of local anesthesia, regardless of the clinical circumstances, are rare (Nichols et al., 2009). In a recent retrospective cohort study, Horwitz and colleagues (2018) used electronic medical record data to assess whether obesity increased the risk of anesthesia-related complications[18] after an aspiration abortion with moderate IV sedation. The study, based in several Massachusetts outpatient clinics, included 20,381 women. Complications were rare and not associated with BMI[19] (Horwitz et al., 2018).

The White and colleagues (2015) systematic review described above identified 11 studies that report patient outcomes related to the use of local anesthesia, moderate sedation, or general anesthesia for aspiration abortions. Anesthesia-related complications were rare regardless of the clinical setting or level of sedation: ≤0.2 percent of office-based procedures and ≤0.5 percent of procedures in surgical centers and hospital-based clinics.

D&E Pain Management

A typical D&E regimen includes a paracervical block supplemented with either moderate sedation (using benzodiazepines and/or opiates) or deep sedation with propofol (without intubation) (NAF, 2017a; RCOG, 2015; WHO, 2012, 2014). In office settings, deep sedation should be used only for healthy patients (ASA I) or patients with mild systemic disease (ASA II), and strict fasting guidelines should be followed before the procedure (ASA Task Force, 2002).

Two large-scale, retrospective analyses have demonstrated the safety of using deep sedation for aspiration and D&E abortions in clinic settings (Dean et al., 2011; Gokhale et al., 2016). Dean and colleagues (2011) assessed the experience of 62,125 women who had an aspiration or D&E abortion (up to 24 weeks' gestation) using deep sedation with propofol

---

[18]The primary outcome assessed was supplemental oxygen administration. Secondary outcomes included reversal agent administration, anesthesia-related adverse events, and intraoperative lowest level of consciousness.

[19]Obesity groups (BMI = 30–34.9; BMI = 35–39.9; BMI ≥40) were compared with women with BMI <25.

(without intubation) in a high-volume licensed clinic in New York State between 2001 and 2008.[20] Deep sedation was provided only to medically eligible patients who followed strict fasting guidelines. The procedures were monitored by an anesthesiologist or CRNA. The researchers reviewed the medical records of all women who were transferred to a hospital (n = 26) because of complications and found that no hospital transfers occurred because of an anesthesia complication.

In a more recent study, Gokhale and colleagues (2016) assessed the outcomes for 5,579 aspiration and D&E abortions using IV sedation (without intubation) at a freestanding abortion clinic in Cleveland from 2012 to 2013. Patients were screened for medical eligibility and followed fasting guidelines. Sedation was administered by registered nurses or by CRNAs if propofol was administered. There were no hospital transfers for anesthesia-related indications. Naloxone was required for opioid reversal in 0.2 percent of patients. The study also compared outcomes for obese and nonobese women; no differences were found.

Induction Pain Management

There is little research on how best to manage pain during an induction (Jackson and Kapp, 2011). Comparisons of different analgesic regimens are not available, and the optimal approach to effective treatment of pain is not well established (Wiebe and Renner, 2014). The options will depend on the provider's resources and the particular clinical circumstances. Nulliparous women may require more analgesia compared with multiparous women (Ashok et al., 2004). The levels of pain in later-gestation induction abortions are said to be similar to those in normal delivery, but the committee found no studies documenting this (Smith et al., 2016; Viviand et al., 2003).

MORTALITY

Death associated with a legal abortion in the United States is an exceedingly rare event. As Table 2-4 shows, the risk of death subsequent to a legal abortion[21] (0.7 per 100,000) is a small fraction of that for childbirth (8.8 per 100,000) (Bartlett et al., 2004; Zane et al., 2015).[22] Abortion-related

---

[20]One patient received an endotracheal intubation.

[21]The CDC defines an abortion-related death as "a death resulting from a direct complication of an induced abortion, an indirect complication caused by a chain of events initiated by an abortion procedure, or the aggravation of a pre-existing condition by the physiologic or psychological effects of the abortion" (Jatlaoui et al., 2016, p. 4).

[22]The CDC calculates the rate of abortion mortality using deaths reported to the CDC Abortion Surveillance System and dividing them by the estimated number of abortion procedures in the United States (CDC, 2017; Jones and Jerman, 2014).

TABLE 2-4 Comparison of Mortality Rates for Abortion, Childbirth, Colonoscopy, Dental Procedures, Plastic Surgery, and Tonsillectomy, United States

Procedure (Study Period)	Mortality Rate (number of deaths per 100,000 procedures)
Abortion (legal) (1988–2010)	0.7
Childbirth (1988–2005)	8.8
Colonoscopy (2001–2015)	2.9
Dental procedures (1999–2005)	0.0 to 1.7
Plastic surgery (2000–2012)	0.8 to 1.7
Tonsillectomy (1968–1972)	2.9 to 6.3

NOTE: Reported tonsillectomy rates were recalculated to reflect the rate per 100,000 procedures.
SOURCES: Baugh et al., 2011; Raymond and Grimes, 2012; Raymond et al., 2014; Reumkens et al., 2016; Zane et al., 2015.

mortality is also lower than that for colonoscopies (2.9 per 100,000), plastic surgery (0.8 to 1.7 per 100,000), dental procedures (0.0 to 1.7 per 100,000), and adult tonsillectomies (2.9 to 6.3 per 100,000). Comparable data for other common medical procedures are difficult to find.

The CDC monitors abortion-related deaths through its Pregnancy Mortality Surveillance System (Jatlaoui et al., 2017). The surveillance data underscore the increased risk of having an abortion later in pregnancy. Zane and colleagues (2015) assessed differences in abortion-related mortality by race, maternal age, and weeks' gestation using data from the CDC surveillance system. Among the 16.1 million legal abortions performed from 1998 to 2010, there were 108 deaths (0.7 per 100,000). Twenty deaths occurred among high-risk women whose pregnancy was life threatening. Infection and anesthesia complications were the most frequent cause of death for procedures performed up to 13 weeks' gestation. After 13 weeks, the deaths reported were due primarily to infection or hemorrhage.

The researchers found that weeks' gestation was the strongest predictor of abortion-related mortality. At 8 weeks' gestation or less, the death rate was 0.3 per 100,000; after 17 weeks, the rate was 6.7 per 100,000. Death rates were approximately three times as high for black women as for white women—similar to the disparities found in pregnancy outcomes overall (Creanga et al., 2012, 2015, 2017; MacDorman et al., 2017). From 2011 to 2013, for example, the overall maternal mortality ratio for non-Hispanic black women was 3.4 times higher than that for non-Hispanic white women (Creanga et al., 2017). A study of maternal mortality in 2013 to 2014 found a 22 percent lower (p = .02) mortality rate for Hispanic women compared with non-Hispanic white women; in 2008–2009, the mortality rate for Hispanic women was similar to that for non-Hispanic white women, but the difference was attributed to the 28 percent increase (p <.001) in mortality for non-Hispanic white women (MacDorman et al., 2017). MacDorman and colleagues (2017) note that almost all of the increase in maternal mortality was among woman aged 40 and older and for nonspecific causes of death.

STATE REGULATION OF ABORTION CARE

States play an essential role in ensuring the safety of health care services, especially through their licensure of clinicians and health care facilities. In every state, clinicians and inpatient facilities (e.g., hospitals, rehabilitation centers) must be licensed by a state board or agency to provide health care services legally (Chaudhry et al., 2013). State licensure may require the facility to be accredited by an independent accrediting organization. Regardless, Medicare and Medicaid, as well as private insurers, require accreditation for inpatient facilities and ASCs to be eligible for reimbursement (CMS, 2012). ASCs provide surgical services to patients not requiring hospitalization when the expected duration of services does not exceed 24 hours (CMS, 2016). In most states, ASCs must also be licensed to provide outpatient surgery, and in many states, ASCs must be accredited (ACFAS, 2017).[23]

Unlike other health care procedures provided in office-based settings, abortions are subject to a wide array of regulations that vary by state. Except for abortion, states typically regulate individual, office-based health services only when the service involves using sedation or general anesthesia (and depending on the level of sedation) (Jones, 2017). Twenty-five states regulate office-based procedures (other than abortion). In 23 of these states,[24] the regulation is triggered by the level of sedation, and in most cases, it requires that the facility be either accredited or licensed by the state in order to offer patients moderate or deep sedation (Jones, 2017; Jones et al., 2018).[25]

State abortion regulations often have a direct impact on the delivery of abortion care. They may stipulate the type of clinician that is allowed to perform an abortion independently of the relevant scope of practice laws

---

[23]According to the American College of Foot and Ankle Surgeons, 46 states require ASCs to be licensed, and 28 states (including the District of Columbia) require accreditation (ACFAS, 2017).

[24]The 23 states are Alabama, Arizona, Arkansas, California, Connecticut, Delaware, Florida, Indiana, Kansas, Louisiana, Mississippi, Nevada, New Jersey, New York, Ohio, Oregon, Pennsylvania, Rhode Island, South Carolina, Tennessee, Texas, Virginia, and Washington.

[25]Personal communication, B. S. Jones, Advancing New Standards in Reproductive Health (ANSIRH), July 3, 2017.

(e.g., qualified advanced practice clinicians [APCs] or physicians without hospital privileges may be barred from performing abortions); how the informed consent process is conducted (e.g., providers may be required to misrepresent the risks of the procedure); the abortion method that is used (e.g., D&Es may be banned); the timing and scheduling of procedures (e.g., women may have to wait 18 to 72 hours after a counseling appointment); the physical attributes of the clinical setting (e.g., procedure room size, corridor width); and other basic elements of care. In most states, the regulations apply to all abortion methods regardless of weeks' gestation, use of sedation, or the invasiveness of the procedure.

See Table 1-1 in Chapter 1 for a listing of abortion-specific regulations by states as of September 1, 2017.

SUMMARY

The clinical evidence presented in this chapter on the provision of safe and high-quality abortion care stands in contrast to the extensive regulatory requirements that state laws impose on the provision of abortion services. These requirements may influence the efficiency of abortion care by requiring medically unnecessary services and multiple visits to the abortion facility, in addition to requiring that care take place in costlier and more sophisticated settings than are clinically necessary. These requirements go beyond the accepted standards of care in the absence of evidence that they improve safety. Some requirements, such as multiple visits and waiting periods, delay abortion services, and by doing so may increase the clinical risks and cost of care. They may also limit women's options for care and impact providers' ability to provide patient-centered care. Furthermore, many of these laws have been documented to reduce the availability of care by imposing unneeded regulations on abortion providers and the settings in which abortion services are delivered. The implications of abortion-specific regulations for the safety and quality of abortion care are described below.

Delaying the Procedure

The clinical evidence makes clear that legal abortions in the United States—whether by medication, aspiration, D&E, or induction—are safe and effective. Serious complications are rare; in the vast majority of studies, they occur in fewer than 1 percent of abortions, and they do not exceed 5 percent in any of the studies the committee identified. However, the risk of a serious complication increases with weeks' gestation. As the number of weeks increases, the invasiveness of the required procedure and the need for deeper levels of sedation also increase. Thus, delaying the abortion increases the risk of harm to the woman.

State regulations that require women to make multiple in-person visits and wait multiple days delay the abortion. If the waiting period is required *after* an in-person counseling appointment, the delay is exacerbated (Roberts et al., 2016; Sanders et al., 2016; White et al., 2017). Restrictions on the types of providers and on the settings in which abortion services can be provided also delay care by reducing the availability of care (Baum et al., 2016; Fuentes et al., 2016; Gerdts et al., 2016; Grossman et al., 2014, 2017).

Financial burdens and difficulty obtaining insurance are frequently cited by women as reasons for delay in obtaining an abortion (Bessett et al., 2011; Drey et al., 2006; Finer et al. 2006; Foster and Kimport, 2013; Foster et al., 2008; French et al., 2016; Janiak et al., 2014; Kiley et al., 2010; Roberts et al., 2014; Upadhyay et al., 2014). As noted in Chapter 1, 33 states prohibit public payers from paying for abortions, and other states have laws that either prohibit health insurance exchange plans (25 states) or private insurance plans (11 states) sold in the state from covering or paying for abortions, with few exceptions.[26]

Counseling and Informed Consent

Long-established ethical and legal standards for informed consent in health care appear to have been compromised in the delivery of abortion care in many areas of the country. Thirty-five states have abortion-specific regulations requiring women to receive counseling before an abortion is performed, and abortion patients in many of these states are offered or given inaccurate or misleading information (verbally or in writing) on reversing medication abortions, risks to future fertility, possible breast cancer risk, and/ or long-term mental health consequences of abortion (Guttmacher Institute, 2017a) (see Table 1-1 in Chapter 1). As noted earlier in this chapter, the principal objective of the informed consent process is that patients understand the nature and risks of the procedure they are considering (AAAHC, 2016; AMA, 2016; HHS, 2017a; Joint Commission, 2016). However, legally requiring providers to inform women about risks that are not supported and are even invalidated by scientific research violates the accepted standards of informed consent. For example, some states require that providers inform women that abortion puts them at greater risk for breast cancer; mental health disorders; and difficulties in having a healthy, successful pregnancy

---

[26]Exceptions are limited and vary by state. They are often made for pregnancies resulting from rape or incest, pregnancies that endanger the woman's life or severely threaten the health of the woman, and cases of fetal impairment.

(Guttmacher Institute, 2017a) (see Table 1-1 in Chapter 1 for a detailed list of states' informed consent requirements). Three states require providers to inform women that a medication abortion can be reversed after the woman takes mifepristone (Guttmacher Institute, 2017a). This information is not supported by research that meets scientific standards. See Chapter 4 for an in-depth review of the long-term health effects of abortion.

Medication Abortion

There is no evidence that the dispensing or taking of mifepristone tablets requires the physical presence of a clinician[27] or a facility with the attributes of an ASC or hospital to ensure safety or quality. The effects of mifepristone occur after women leave the clinic, and extensive research shows that serious complications are rare. The risks of medication abortion are similar in magnitude to the risks of taking commonly prescribed and over-the-counter medications such as antibiotics and NSAIDs. In 35 states, however, only physicians are permitted to give women the mifepristone tablet(s) required to begin the process of medication abortion (RHN, 2017). In 19 states, the clinician (a physician or other provider if allowed) must be physically present to provide the medication, thus prohibiting the use of telemedicine to prescribe the medication remotely for abortion (Guttmacher Institute, 2017b). In 17 states, medication abortions must be performed in a facility that meets the structural standards of ASCs even though the abortion will occur outside the clinical setting, and there is no evidence to suggest that these regulations improve safety or quality.

Aspiration Abortions

Aspirations are minimally invasive and commonly used for a variety of purposes in gynecology practices, including for early pregnancy loss (miscarriage). Aspiration abortions are performed safely in office-based settings and can be provided by appropriately trained APCs, as well as family practice physicians and OB/GYNs. If moderate sedation is used, the procedure should be performed in a facility that meets the relevant ASA facility standards. There is no evidence that performing aspiration abortions in ASCs increases the safety or efficacy of the procedure. The state regulations described above also affect aspiration abortion procedures: 44 states do not allow APCs to perform aspirations, and 16 states mandate that the procedure be performed in an ASC-like facility.

---

[27]Chapter 3 reviews the clinical competencies needed to provide safe and high-quality abortions, as well as state regulations regarding the role of APCs.

D&E and Induction Abortions

D&E is usually the medically preferred method for abortions at 14 weeks' gestation or later. The alternative—induction—is more painful, slower, and more expensive. D&Es are banned in Mississippi[28] and West Virginia[29] except if the woman's physical health or life is severely threatened.

REFERENCES

AAAHC (Accreditation Association for Ambulatory Health Care). 2016. *Informed consent.* https://www.aaahc.org/Global/Newsletter_Connection/2016Jul_Connection_FINAL.pdf (accessed September 25, 2017).

AANA (American Association of Nurse Anesthetists). 2016. *Informed consent in anesthesia. Policy and practice considerations.* https://www.aana.com/docs/default-source/practice-aana-com-web-documents-(all)/informed-consent-for-anesthesia-care.pdf (accessed January 23, 2018).

ACFAS (American College of Foot and Ankle Surgeons). 2017. *Ambulatory surgical centers: Regulation and accreditation.* https://www.acfas.org/Physicians/content.aspx?id=628 (accessed November 28, 2017).

ACOG (American College of Obstetricians and Gynecologists). 2013. ACOG practice bulletin 135: Second-trimester abortion. *Obstetrics & Gynecology* 121(6):1394–1406.

ACOG. 2015. *Committee opinion number 439 (reaffirmed). Informed consent.* https://www.acog.org/-/media/Committee-Opinions/Committee-on-Ethics/co439.pdf?dmc=1&ts=20171018T1431178490 (accessed August 1, 2017).

ACOG. 2017a. *About us.* https://www.acog.org/About-ACOG/About-Us (accessed August 23, 2017).

ACOG. 2017b. *Practice bulletin 186: Long-acting reversible contraception: Implants and intrauterine devices.* https://www.acog.org/Resources-And-Publications/Practice-Bulletins/Committee-on-Practice-Bulletins-Gynecology/Long-Acting-Reversible-Contraception-Implants-and-Intrauterine-Devices (accessed October 30, 2017).

ACOG and SFP (Society for Family Planning). 2014. Practice bulletin 143: Medical management of first-trimester abortion. *Obstetrics & Gynecology* 123(3):676–692.

Aiken, A. R. A., K. A. Guthrie, M. Schellekens, J. Trussell, and R. Gomperts. 2018. Barriers to accessing abortion services and perspectives on using mifepristone and misoprostol at home in Great Britain. *Contraception* 97(2):177–183. doi:10.1016/j.contraception.2017.09.003.

Allen, R. H., and A. B. Goldberg. 2016. Cervical dilation before first-trimester surgical abortion (<14 weeks' gestation). *Contraception* 93(4):277–291.

Allen, R. H., J. Fortin, D. Bartz, A. B. Goldberg, and M. A. Clark. 2012. Women's preferences for pain control during first-trimester surgical abortion: A qualitative study. *Contraception* 85(4):413–418.

Allen, R. H., E. Micks, and A. Edelman. 2013. Pain relief for obstetric and gynecologic ambulatory procedures. *Obstetrics & Gynecology Clinics of North America* 40(4):625–645.

---

[28]Mississippi Unborn Child Protection from Dismemberment Abortion Act, Mississippi HB 519, Reg. Sess. 2015–2016 (2016).

[29]Unborn Child Protection from Dismemberment Abortion Act, West Virginia SB 10, Reg. Sess. 2015–2016 (2016).

AMA (American Medical Association). 2016. *Chapter 2: Opinions on consent, communication, and decision making. Code of medical ethics.* Washington, DC: American Medical Association. https://www.ama-assn.org/sites/default/files/media-browser/code-of-medical-ethics-chapter-2.pdf (accessed February 22, 2018).

Ames, C. M., and W. V. Norman. 2012. Preventing repeat abortion in Canada: Is the immediate insertion of intrauterine devices postabortion a cost-effective option associated with fewer repeat abortions? *Contraception* 85(1):1–5.

ANSIRH (Advancing New Standards in Reproductive Health). 2017. *Abortion facility standards initiative.* https://www.ansirh.org/research/abortion-facility-standards-initiative (accessed October 24, 2017).

ASA (American Society of Anesthesiologists). 2013. *Statement on nonoperating room anesthetizing locations.* http://www.asahq.org/~/media/Sites/ASAHQ/Files/Public/Resources/standards-guidelines/statement-on-nonoperating-room-anesthetizing-locations.pdf (accessed October 4, 2017).

ASA. 2014a. *ASA physical status classification system.* https://www.asahq.org/resources/clinical-information/asa-physical-status-classification-system# (accessed October 5, 2017).

ASA. 2014b. *Guidelines for office-based anesthesia (reaffirmed).* https://www.asahq.org/~/media/sites/asahq/files/public/resources/standards-guidelines/guidelines-for-office-based-anesthesia.pdf (accessed July 2, 2017).

ASA. 2015. *Standards for basic anesthetic monitoring (reaffirmed).* http://www.asahq.org/sitecore/shell/~/media/sites/asahq/files/public/resources/publications/epubs/standards-for-basic-anesthetic-monitoring-epub.epub (accessed July 10, 2017).

ASA Committee on Ethics. 2016. *Frequently asked questions on informed consent for procedures.* Version 1.5 (draft document). http://www.asahq.org/~/media/sites/asahq/files/public/resources/faq-anesthesia-consent-ver-1-5.pdf (accessed July 31, 2017).

ASA Task Force on Sedation and Analgesia by Non-Anesthesiologists. 2002. Practice guidelines for sedation and analgesia by non-anesthesiologists. *Anesthesiology* 96(4):1004–1017.

Ashok, P. W., A. Templeton, P. T. Wagaarachchi, and G. M. Flett. 2002. Factors affecting the outcome of early medical abortion: A review of 4,132 consecutive cases. *British Journal of Obstetrics & Gynaecology* 109(11):1281–1289.

Ashok, P. W., A. Templeton, P. T. Wagaarachchi, and G. M. Flett. 2004. Midtrimester medical termination of pregnancy: A review of 1002 consecutive cases. *Contraception* 69(1):51–58.

Autry, A. M., E. C. Hayes, G. F. Jacobson, and R. S. Kirby. 2002. A comparison of medical induction and dilation and evacuation for second-trimester abortion. *American Journal of Obstetrics and Gynecology* 187(2):393–397.

Baker, A., and T. Beresford. 2009. Chapter 5. Informed consent, patient education, and counseling. In *Management of unintended and abnormal pregnancy: Comprehensive abortion care*, edited by M. Paul, E. S. Lichtenberg, L. Borgatta, D. A. Grimes, P. G. Stubblefield and M. D. Creinin. Hoboken, NJ: Wiley-Blackwell. Pp. 48–62.

Baron, C., S. Cameron, and A. Johnstone. 2015. Do women seeking termination of pregnancy need pre-abortion counselling? *Journal of Family Planning and Reproductive Health Care* 41(3):181–185.

Bartlett, L. A., C. J. Berg, H. B. Shulman, S. B. Zane, C. A. Green, S. Whitehead, and H. K. Atrash. 2004. Risk factors for legal induced abortion-related mortality in the United States. *Obstetrics and Gynecology* 103(4):729–737.

Bassi, C., B. Langer, and G. Schlaeder. 1994. Legal abortion by menstrual regulation: A report of 778 cases. *Journal of Obstetrics and Gynaecology* 14(3):175–179.

Baugh, R. F., S. M. Archer, R. B. Mitchell, R. M. Rosenfeld, R. Amin, J. J. Burns, D. H. Darrow, T. Giordano, R. S. Litman, K. K. Li, M. E. Mannix, R. H. Schwartz, G. Setzen, E. R. Wald, E. Wall, G. Sandberg, and M. M. Patel. 2011. Clinical practice guideline: Tonsillectomy in children. *Otolaryngology—Head & Neck Surgery* 144(1 Suppl.):S1–S30.
Baum, S. E., K. White, K. Hopkins, J. E. Potter, and D. Grossman. 2016. Women's experience obtaining abortion care in Texas after implementation of restrictive abortion laws: A qualitative study. *PLoS One* 11(10):e0165048.
Ben-Ami, I., D. Schneider, R. Svirsky, N. Smorgick, M. Pansky, and R. Halperin. 2009. Safety of late second-trimester pregnancy termination by laminaria dilatation and evacuation in patients with previous multiple cesarean sections. *American Journal of Obstetrics and Gynecology* 201:154.e1–5.
Benson, L., E. A. Micks, C. Ingalls, and S. W. Prager. 2016. Safety of outpatient surgical abortion for obese patients in the first and second trimesters. *Obstetrics & Gynecology* 128(5):1065–1070.
Berghella, V., J. Airoldi, A. M. O'Neill, K. Einhorn, and M. Hoffman. 2009. Misoprostol for second trimester pregnancy termination in women with prior caesarean: A systematic review. *BJOG: An International Journal of Obstetrics & Gynaecology* 116(9):1151–1157.
Bessett, D., K. Gorski, D. Jinadasa, M. Ostrow, and M. J. Peterson. 2011. Out of time and out of pocket: Experiences of women seeking state-subsidized insurance for abortion care in Massachusetts. *Women's Health Issues* 21(3 Suppl.):S21–S25.
Borgatta, L. 2011. *Labor induction termination of pregnancy.* https://www.glowm.com/section_view/heading/Labor%20Induction%20Termination%20of%20Pregnancy/item/443 (accessed September 13, 2017).
Borkowski, L., J. Strasser, A. Allina, and S. Wood. 2015. *Medication abortion. Overview of research & policy in the United States.* http://publichealth.gwu.edu/sites/default/files/Medication_Abortion_white_paper.pdf (accessed January 25, 2017).
Bourassa, D., and J. Berube. 2007. The prevalence of intimate partner violence among women and teenagers seeking abortion compared with those continuing pregnancy. *Journal of Obstetrics and Gynaecology Canada* 29(5):415–423.
Bracken, H., W. Clark, E. S. Lichtenberg, S. M. Schweikert, J. Tanenhaus, A. Barajas, L. Alpert, and B. Winikoff. 2011. Alternatives to routine ultrasound for eligibility assessment prior to early termination of pregnancy with mifepristone-misoprostol. *BJOG: An International Journal of Obstetrics & Gynaecology* 118(1):17–23.
Brown, S. 2013. Is counselling necessary? Making the decision to have an abortion. A qualitative interview study. *The European Journal of Contraception & Reproductive Health Care* 18(1):44–48.
Bryant, A. G., D. A. Grimes, J. M. Garrett, and G. S. Stuart. 2011. Second-trimester abortion for fetal anomalies or fetal death: Labor induction compared with dilation and evacuation. *Obstetrics & Gynecology* 117(4):788–792.
Cates, Jr., W., K. F. Schulz, D. A. Grimes, A. J. Horowitz, F. A. Lyon, F. H. Kravitz, and M. J. Frisch. 1982. Dilation and evacuation procedures and second-trimester abortions. The role of physician skill and hospital setting. *Journal of the American Medical Association* 248(5):559–563.
Cates, Jr., W., K. F. Schulz, and D. A. Grimes. 1983. The risks associated with teenage abortion. *New England Journal of Medicine* 309(11):621–624.
CDC (Centers for Disease Control and Prevention). 2017. *Pregnancy Mortality Surveillance System.* https://www.cdc.gov/reproductivehealth/maternalinfanthealth/pmss.html (accessed November 1, 2017).
CDER (Center for Drug Evaluation and Review). 2016. *Application number: 020687Orig1s020. Medical review(s).* https://www.accessdata.fda.gov/drugsatfda_docs/nda/2016/020687Orig1s020MedR.pdf (accessed April 24, 2017).

Chai, J., C. Y. Wong, and P. C. Ho. 2013. A randomized clinical trial comparing the short-term side effects of sublingual and buccal routes of misoprostol administration for medical abortions up to 63 days' gestation. *Contraception* 87(4):480–485.

Chaudhry, H. J., F. E. Cain, M. A. Staz, L. A. Talmage, J. A. Rhyne, and J. V. Thomas. 2013. The evidence and rationale for maintenance of licensure. *Journal of Medical Regulation* 99(1):19–26.

Chen, M. J., and M. D. Creinin. 2015. Mifepristone with buccal misoprostol for medical abortion: A systematic review. *Obstetrics & Gynecology* 126(1):12–21.

Chong, E., L. J. Frye, J. Castle, G. Dean, L. Kuehl, and B. Winikoff. 2015. A prospective, non-randomized study of home use of mifepristone for medical abortion in the U.S. *Contraception* 92(3):215–219.

Clark, W. H., D. Hassoun, K. Gemzell-Danielsson, C. Fiala, and B. Winikoff. 2005. Home use of two doses of misoprostol after mifepristone for medical abortion: A pilot study in Sweden and France. *European Journal of Contraception & Reproductive Health Care* 10(3):184–191.

Cleland, K., M. D. Creinin, D. Nucatola, M. Nshom, and J. Trussell. 2013. Significant adverse events and outcomes after medical abortion. *Obstetrics & Gynecology* 121(1):166–171.

CMS (Centers for Medicare & Medicaid Services). 2012. Medicare and Medicaid programs reform of hospital and critical access hospital conditions of participation. *Federal Register* 77(95):29034–29040.

CMS. 2016. *Ambulatory Surgery Centers.* https://www.cms.gov/Medicare/Provider-Enrollment-and-Certification/CertificationandComplianc/ASCs.html (accessed November 10, 2017).

Conkling, K., C. Karki, H. Tuladhar, H. Bracken, and B. Winikoff. 2015. A prospective open-label study of home use of mifepristone for medical abortion in Nepal. *International Journal of Gynaecology & Obstetrics* 128(3):220–223.

Constant, D., J. Harries, T. Malaba, L. Myer, M. Patel, G. Petro, and D. Grossman. 2016. Clinical outcomes and women's experiences before and after the introduction of mifepristone into second-trimester medical abortion services in South Africa. *PLoS One* 11(9):e0161843.

Creanga, A. A., C. J. Berg, C. Syverson, K. Seed, F. C. Bruce, and W. M. Callaghan. 2012. Race, ethnicity, and nativity differentials in pregnancy-related mortality in the United States: 1993–2006. *Obstetrics & Gynecology* 125(1):5–12.

Creanga, A. A., C. J. Berg, C. Syverson, K. Seed, F. C. Bruce, and W. M. Callaghan. 2015. Pregnancy-related mortality in the United States, 2006–2010. *Obstetrics & Gynecology* 120(2):261–268.

Creanga, A. A., C. Syverson, K. Seed, and W. M. Callaghan. 2017. Pregnancy-related mortality in the United States, 2011–2013. *Obstetrics & Gynecology* 130(2):366–373.

Dabrowska, A. 2017. *FDA Risk Evaluation and Mitigation Strategies (REMS): Description and effect on generic drug development.* Washington, DC: Congressional Research Service.

Darney, P. D., and R. L. Sweet. 1989. Routine intraoperative ultrasonography for second trimester abortion reduces incidence of uterine perforation. *Journal of Ultrasound in Medicine* 8(2):71–75.

Dean, G., A. R. Jacobs, R. C. Goldstein, C. M. Gevirtz, and M. E. Paul. 2011. The safety of deep sedation without intubation for abortion in the outpatient setting. *Journal of Clinical Anesthesia* 23(6):437–442.

Delgado, G., and M. L. Davenport. 2012. Progesterone use to reverse the effects of mifepristone. *Annals of Pharmacotherapy* 46:e36.

Diedrich, J. T., T. Madden, Q. Zhao, and J. F. Peipert. 2015. Long-term utilization and continuation of intrauterine devices. *American Journal of Obstetrics and Gynecology* 213(5):662.e1–662.e8.

Dragoman, M. V., D. Grossman, N. Kapp, N. M. Huong, N. Habib, D. L. Dung, and A. Tamang. 2016. Two prophylactic medication approaches in addition to a pain control regimen for early medical abortion <63 days' gestation with mifepristone and misoprostol: Study protocol for a randomized, controlled trial. *Reproductive Health* 13(1):132. doi:10.1186/s12978-016-0246-5.

Drey, E. A., D. G. Foster, R. A. Jackson, S. J. Lee, L. H. Cardenas, and P. D. Darney. 2006. Risk factors associated with presenting for abortion in the second trimester. *Obstetrics & Gynecology* 107(1):128–135.

Edelman, A., M. D. Nichols, and J. Jensen. 2001. Comparison of pain and time of procedures with two first-trimester abortion techniques performed by residents and faculty. *American Journal of Obstetrics and Gynecology* 184(7):1564–1567.

Evins, G., and N. Chescheir. 1996. Prevalence of domestic violence among women seeking abortion services. *Women's Health Issues* 6(4):204–210.

Fanslow, J., M. Silva, A. Whitehead, and E. Robinson. 2008. Pregnancy outcomes and intimate partner violence in New Zealand. *Australian and New Zealand Journal of Obstetrics and Gynecology* 48(4):391–397.

FDA (U.S. Food and Drug Administration). 2011. *Mifepristone U.S. postmarketing adverse events summary through 04/30/2011.* http://wayback.archive-it.org/7993/20161024033523/http://www.fda.gov/downloads/Drugs/DrugSafety/PostmarketDrugSafetyInformationforPatientsandProviders/UCM263353.pdf (accessed February 5, 2018).

FDA. 2016a. *FDA label: Mifeprex.* Reference ID: 3909592. https://www.accessdata.fda.gov/drugsatfda_docs/label/2016/020687s020lbl.pdf (accessed March 10, 2017).

FDA. 2016b. *Highlights of prescribing information. Mifeprex (revised 3/2016).* https://www.fda.gov/drugs/drugsafety/postmarketdrugsafetyinformationforpatientsandproviders/ucm111323.htm (accessed May 31, 2017).

FDA. 2016c. *Questions and answers on Mifeprex.* https://www.fda.gov/drugs/drugsafety/postmarketdrugsafetyinformationforpatientsandproviders/ucm492705.htm (accessed August 10, 2017).

Fiala, C., B. Winikoff, L. Helstrom, M. Hellborg, and K. Gemzell-Danielsson. 2004. Acceptability of home-use of misoprostol in medical abortion. *Contraception* 70(5):387–392.

Finer, L. B., L. F. Frohwirth, L. A. Dauphinee, S. Singh, and A. M. Moore. 2006. Timing of steps and reasons for delays in obtaining abortions in the United States. *Contraception* 74(4):334–344.

Fisher, W. A., S. S. Singh, P. A. Shuper, M. Carey, F. Otchet, D. MacLean-Brine, D. Dal Bello, and J. Gunter. 2005. Characteristics of women undergoing repeat induced abortion. *Canadian Medical Journal* 172(5):637–641.

Fleisher, L. A., L. R. Pasternak, and A. Lyles. 2007. A novel index of elevated risk of inpatient hospital admission immediately following outpatient surgery. *Archives of Surgery* 142(3):263–268.

Foster, D. G., and K. Kimport. 2013. Who seeks abortions at or after 20 weeks? *Perspectives on Sexual and Reproductive Health* 45(4):210–218.

Foster, D. G., R. A. Jackson, K. Cosby, T. A. Weitz, P. D. Darney, and E. A. Drey. 2008. Predictors of delay in each step leading to an abortion. *Contraception* 77(4):289–293.

Fox, M. C., J. Oat-Judge, K. Severson, R. M. Jamshidi, R. H. Singh, R. McDonald-Mosley, and A. E. Burke. 2011. Immediate placement of intrauterine devices after first and second trimester pregnancy termination. *Contraception* 83(1):34–40.

French, V., R. Anthony, C. Souder, C. Geistkemper, E. Drey, and J. Steinauer. 2016. Influence of clinician referral on Nebraska women's decision-to-abortion time. *Contraception* 93(3):236–243.

Frick, A. C., E. A. Drey, J. T. Diedrich, and J. E. Steinauer. 2010. Effect of prior cesarean delivery on risk of second-trimester surgical abortion complications. *Obstetrics & Gynecology* 115(4):760–764.

Fuentes, L., S. Lebenkoff, K. White, C. Gerdts, K. Hopkins, J. E. Potter, and D. Grossman. 2016. Women's experiences seeking abortion care shortly after the closure of clinics due to a restrictive law in Texas. *Contraception* 93(4):292–297.

Gassman, A. L., C. P. Nguyen, and H. V. Joffe. 2017. FDA regulation of prescription drugs. *New England Journal of Medicine* 376(7):674–682.

Gemzell-Danielsson, K., and S. Lalitkumar. 2008. Second trimester medical abortion with mifepristone-misoprostol and misoprostol alone: A review of methods and management. *Reproductive Health Matters* 16(31 Suppl.):162–172.

Gerdts, C., L. Fuentes, D. Grossman, K. White, B. Keefe-Oates, S. E. Baum, K. Hopkins, C. W. Stolp, and J. E. Potter. 2016. Impact of clinic closures on women obtaining abortion services after implementation of a restrictive law in Texas. *American Journal of Public Health* 106(5):857–864.

Gissler, M., E. Karalis, and V. M. Ulander. 2015. Decreased suicide rate after induced abortion, after the current care guidelines in Finland 1987–2012. *Scandinavian Journal of Public Health* 43(1):99–101.

Glander, S. S., M. L. Moore, R. Michielutte, and L. H. Parsons. 1998. The prevalence of domestic violence among women seeking abortion. *Obstetrics & Gynecology* 91(6):1002–1006.

Goh, S. E., and K. J. Thong. 2006. Induction of second trimester abortion (12–20 weeks) with mifepristone and misoprostol: A review of 386 consecutive cases. *Contraception* 73(5):516–519.

Gokhale, P., J. R. Lappen, J. H. Waters, and L. K. Perriera. 2016. Intravenous sedation without intubation and the risk of anesthesia complications for obese and non-obese women undergoing surgical abortion: A retrospective cohort study. *Anesthesia & Analgesia* 122(6):1957–1962.

Goldberg, A. B., G. Dean, M. S. Kang, S. Youssof, and P. D. Darney. 2004. Manual versus electric vacuum aspiration for early first-trimester abortion: A controlled study of complication rates. *Obstetrics & Gynecology* 103(1):101–107.

Goldstein, S. R., and M. F. Reeves. 2009. Chapter 6. Clinical assessment and ultrasound in early pregnancy. In *Management of unintended and abnormal pregnancy: Comprehensive abortion care*, edited by M. Paul, E. S. Lichtenberg, L. Borgatta, D. A. Grimes, P. G. Stubblefield, and M. D. Creinin. Hoboken, NJ: Wiley-Blackwell. Pp. 157–177.

Goodman, S., S. K. Hendlish, M. F. Reeves, and A. Foster-Rosales. 2008. Impact of immediate postabortal insertion of intrauterine contraception on repeat abortion. *Contraception* 78:143–148.

Goodman, S., G. Flaxman, and the TEACH Trainers Collaborative Working Group. 2016. *Early Abortion Training Workbook*, 4th ed. San Francisco, CA: Bixby Center for Global Reproductive Health.

Gouk, E. V., K. Lincoln, A. Khair, J. Haslock, J. Knight, and D. J. Cruickshank. 1999. Medical termination of pregnancy at 63 to 83 days gestation. *British Journal of Obstetrics & Gynaecology* 106(6):535–539.

Goyal, V. 2009. Uterine rupture in second-trimester misoprostol-induced abortion after cesarean delivery: A systematic review. *Obstetrics & Gynecology* 113(5):1117–1123.

Goyal, V., C. Canfield, A. R. A. Aiken, A. Dermish, and J. E. Potter. 2017. Postabortion contraceptive use and continuation when long-acting reversible contraception is free. *Obstetrics & Gynecology* 129(4):655–662.

Graham, R. 2017. A new front in the war over reproductive rights: Abortion-pill reversal. *The New York Times*, July 18.

Grimes, D. A., K. F. Schulz, W. Cates, Jr., and C. W. Tyler, Jr. 1977. Mid-trimester abortion by dilation and evacuation: A safe and practical alternative. *New England Journal of Medicine* 296(20):1141–1145.

Grimes, D. A., S. M. Smith, and A. D. Witham. 2004. Mifepristone and misoprostol versus dilation and evacuation for midtrimester abortion: A pilot randomised controlled trial. *British Journal of Obstetrics & Gynaecology* 111(2):148–153.

Grimes, D. A., L. M. Lopez, K. F. Schulz, and N. L. Stanwood. 2010. Immediate post-abortal insertion of intrauterine devices. *Cochrane Database of Systematic Reviews* 16(6):CD001777.

Grossman, D., and K. Grindlay. 2017. Safety of medical abortion provided through tele-medicine compared with in person. *Obstetrics & Gynecology* 130(4):778–782.

Grossman, D., K. Blanchard, and P. Blumenthal. 2008. Complications after second trimester surgical and medical abortion. *Reproductive Health Matters* 16(31 Suppl.):173–182.

Grossman, D., K. Grindlay, T. Buchacker, K. Lane, and K. Blanchard. 2011a. Effectiveness and acceptability of medical abortion provided through telemedicine. *Obstetrics & Gynecology* 118(2 Pt. 1):296–303.

Grossman, D., D. Constant, N. Lince, M. Alblas, K. Blanchard, and J. Harries. 2011b. Surgi-cal and medical second trimester abortion in South Africa: A cross-sectional study. *BMC Health Services Research* 11(224):1–9.

Grossman, D. A., K. Grindlay, T. Buchacker, J. E. Potter, and C. P. Schmertmann. 2013. Changes in service delivery patterns after introduction of telemedicine provision of medi-cal abortion in Iowa. *American Journal of Public Health* 103(1):73–78.

Grossman, D., S. Baum, L. Fuentes, K. White, K. Hopkins, A. Stevenson, and J. E. Potter. 2014. Change in abortion services after implementation of a restrictive law in Texas. *Contraception* 90(5):496–501.

Grossman, D., K. White, L. Harris, M. Reeves, P. D. Blumenthal, B. Winikoff, and D. A. Grimes. 2015. Continuing pregnancy after mifepristone and "reversal" of first-trimester medical abortion: A systematic review. *Contraception* 92(3):206–211.

Grossman, D., K. White, K. Hopkins, and J. E. Potter. 2017. Change in distance to nearest facility and abortion in Texas, 2012 to 2014. *Journal of the American Medical Associa-tion* 317(4):437–438.

Guengant, J. P., J. Bangou, B. Elul, and C. Ellertson. 1999. Mifepristone-misoprostol medi-cal abortion: Home administration of misoprostol in Guadeloupe. *Contraception* 60(3):167–172.

Guiahi, M., G. Schiller, J. Sheeder, and S. Teal. 2015. Safety of first-trimester uterine evacua-tion in the outpatient setting for women with common chronic conditions. *Contraception* 92(5):453–457.

Guttmacher Institute. 2017a. *Counseling and waiting periods for abortion.* https://www.guttmacher.org/print/state-policy/explore/counseling-and-waiting-periods-abortion (ac-cessed November 1, 2017).

Guttmacher Institute. 2017b. *Medication abortion.* https://www.guttmacher.org/print/state-policy/explore/medication-abortion (accessed September 12, 2017).

Guyatt, G. H., A. D. Oxman, G. Vist, R. Kunz, J. Brozek, P. Alonso-Coello, V. Montori, E. A. Akl, B. Djulbegovic, Y. Falck-Ytter, S. L. Norris, J. W. Williams, Jr., D. Atkins, J. Meerpohl, and H. J. Schünemann. 2011. GRADE guidelines: 4. Rating the quality of evidence—study limitations (risk of bias). *Journal of Clinical Epidemiology* 64(4):407–415.

Hammond, C., and S. Chasen. 2009. Chapter 11. Dilation and evacuation. In *Management of unintended and abnormal pregnancy: Comprehensive abortion care*, edited by M. Paul, E. S. Lichtenberg, L. Borgatta, D. A. Grimes, P. G. Stubblefield, and M. D. Creinin. Hoboken, NJ: Wiley-Blackwell. Pp. 157–177.

Hamoda, H., P. W. Ashok, G. M. Flett, and A. Templeton. 2003. Medical abortion at 64 to 91 days of gestation: A review of 483 consecutive cases. *American Journal of Obstetrics and Gynecology* 188(5):1315–1319.

Hawkey, C. J., and M. J. Langman. 2003. Non-steroidal anti-inflammatory drugs: Overall risks and management. Complementary roles for COX-2 inhibitors and proton pump inhibitors. *Gut* 52(4):600–608.

Hern, W. M. 2016. *Second-trimester surgical abortion.* https://www.glowm.com/section_view/heading/Second-Trimester%20Surgical%20Abortion/item/441 (accessed October 6, 2017).

HHS (U.S. Department of Health and Human Services). 2017a. Potential inclusion of the quality of informed consent documents for hospital-performed, elective procedures measure. *Federal Register* 82(155):38362–38363.

HHS. 2017b. *Telemedicine.* https://www.medicaid.gov/medicaid/benefits/telemed/index.html (accessed November 10, 2017).

Hirschhorn, L. R., Y. Trnka, A. Onderdonk, M. L. Lee, and R. Platt. 1994. Epidemiology of community-acquired clostridium difficile-associated diarrhea. *Journal of Infectious Disease* 169(1):127–133.

Hognert, H., H. K. Kallner, S. Cameron, C. Nyrelli, I. Jawad, R. Heller, A. Aronsson, I. Lindh, L. Benson, and K. Gemzell-Danielsson. 2016. Immediate versus delayed insertion of an etonogestrel releasing implant at medical abortion—a randomized controlled equivalence trial. *Human Reproduction* 31(11):2484–2490.

Horwitz, G., D. Roncari, K. P. Braaten, R. Maurer, J. Fortin, and A. B. Goldberg. 2018. Moderate intravenous sedation for first trimester surgical abortion: A comparison of adverse outcomes between obese and normal-weight women. *Contraception* 97(1):48–53.

Ibis Reproductive Health. 2015. *Clinical research standards.* http://laterabortion.org/clinical-research-standards (accessed October 6, 2017).

IOM (Institute of Medicine). 2001. *Crossing the quality chasm: A new health system for the 21st century.* Washington, DC: National Academy Press.

Ireland, L. D., M. Gatter, and A. Y. Chen. 2015. Medical compared with surgical abortion for effective pregnancy termination in the first trimester. *Obstetrics & Gynecology* 126(1):22–28.

Jackson, E., and N. Kapp. 2011. Pain control in first-trimester and second-trimester medical termination of pregnancy: A systematic review. *Contraception* 83(2):116–126.

Jacot, F. R. M., C. Poulin, A. P. Bilodeau, M. Morin, S. Moreau, F. Gendron, and D. Mercier. 1993. A five-year experience with second-trimester induced abortions: No increase in complication rate as compared to the first trimester. *American Journal of Obstetrics and Gynecology* 168(2):633–637.

Janiak, E., I. Kawachi, A. Goldberg, and B. Gottlieb. 2014. Abortion barriers and perceptions of gestational age among women seeking abortion care in the latter half of the second trimester. *Contraception* 89(4):322–327.

Janssen, P. A., V. L. Holt, N. K. Sugg, I. Emanuel, C. M. Critchlow, and A. D. Henderson. 2003. Intimate partner violence and adverse pregnancy outcomes: A population-based study. *American Journal of Obstetrics and Gynecology* 188(5):1341–1347.

Jatlaoui, T. C., A. Ewing, M. G. Mandel, K. B. Simmons, D. B. Suchdev, D. J. Jamieson, and K. Pazol. 2016. Abortion surveillance—United States, 2013. *MMWR Surveillance Summaries* 65(12):1–44.

Jatlaoui, T., J. Shah, M. G. Mandel, K. W. Krashin, D. B. Suchdev, D. J. Jamieson, and K. Pazol. 2017. Abortion surveillance—United States, 2014. *Morbidity and Mortality Weekly Reports* 66(SS-24):1–48.

Jerman, J., R. K. Jones, and T. Onda. 2016. *Characteristics of U.S. abortion patients in 2014 and changes since 2008.* https://www.guttmacher.org/sites/default/files/report_pdf/characteristics-us-abortion-patients-2014.pdf (accessed October 17, 2016).

Joint Commission. 2016. Informed consent: More than getting a signature. *QuickSafety. An Advisory on Safety & Quality Issues* 21(1–3).

Joint Commission Resources. 2016. *Resource guide. Centers for Medicare & Medicaid Services (CMS)—Complying with CMS Conditions of Participation (CoP) §482.51: Surgical services.* http://4562.cmssurg.qualityandsafetynetwork.com/downloads/16_JCR6_4562.pdf (accessed September 25, 2017).

Jones, B. S. 2017. *Facility standards for abortions and other outpatient procedures.* Presentation to the Committee on Reproductive Health: Assessing the Safety and Quality of Abortion Care in the U.S. (Health and Medicine Division of the National Academies of Sciences, Engineering, and Medicine). Workshop on Facility Standards and the Safety of Outpatient Procedures, March 24, Washington, DC.

Jones, B. S., S. Daniel, and L. K. Cloud. 2018. State law approaches to facility regulation of abortion and other office interventions. *American Journal of Public Health.* doi: 10.2105/AJPH.2017.304278.

Jones, R. K., and J. Jerman. 2014. Abortion incidence and service availability in the United States, 2011. *Perspectives on Sexual and Reproductive Health* 46(1):3–14.

Jones, R. K., and J. Jerman. 2017. Abortion incidence and service availability in the United States, 2014. *Perspectives on Sexual and Reproductive Health* 49(1):1–11.

Kaneshiro, B., A. Edelman, R. K. Sneeringer, and R. G. Ponce de Leon. 2011. Expanding medical abortion: Can medical abortion be effectively provided without the routine use of ultrasound? *Contraception* 83(3):194–201.

Kapp, N., L. Borgatta, P. Stubblefield, O. Vragovic, and N. Moreno. 2007. Mifepristone in second-trimester medical abortion: A randomized controlled trial. *Obstetrics & Gynecology* 110(6):1304–1310.

Keeling, J., L. Birch, and P. Green. 2004. Pregnancy counselling clinic: A questionnaire survey of intimate partner abuse. *Journal of Family Planning & Reproductive Health Care* 30(3):156–158.

Kelly, T., J. Suddes, D. Howel, J. Hewison, and S. Robson. 2010. Comparing medical versus surgical termination of pregnancy at 13–20 weeks of gestation: A randomised controlled trial. *British Journal of Obstetrics & Gynaecology* 117(12):1512–1520.

Kilander, H., S. Alehagen, L. Svedlund, K. Westlund, J. Thor, and J. Brynhildsen. 2016. Likelihood of repeat abortion in a Swedish cohort according to the choice of post-abortion contraception: A longitudinal study. *Acta Obstetricia et Gynecologica Scandinavica* 95(5):565–571.

Kiley, J. W., L. M. Yee, C. M. Niemi, J. M. Feinglass, and M. A. Simon. 2010. Delays in request for pregnancy termination: Comparison of patients in the first and second trimesters. *Contraception* 81(5):446–451.

Kinnersley, P., K. Phillips, K. Savage, M. J. Kelly, E. Farrell, B. Morgan, R. Whistance, V. Lewis, M. K. Mann, B. L. Stephens, and J. Blazeby. 2013. Interventions to promote informed consent for patients undergoing surgical and other invasive healthcare procedures. *Cochrane Database of Systematic Reviews* 7:20137CD009445.

Kulier, R., N. Kapp, A. M. Gulmezoglu, G. J. Hofmeyr, L. Cheng, and A Campana. 2011. Medical methods for first trimester abortion. *Cochrane Database of Systematic Reviews* (11):CD002855.

Lederle, L., J. E. Steinauer, A. Montgomery, S. Aksel, E. A. Drey, and J. L. Kerns. 2015. Obesity as a risk factor for complications after second-trimester abortion by dilation and evacuation. *Obstetrics & Gynecology* 126(3):585–592.

Leung, T. W., W. C. Leung, P. L. Chang, and P. C. Ho. 2002. A comparison of the prevalence of domestic violence between patients seeking termination of pregnancy and other general gynecology patients. *International Journal of Gynaecology & Obstetrics* 77(1):47–54.

Livshits, A., R. Machtinger, L. B. David, M. Spira, A. Moshe-Zahav, and D. S. Seidman. 2009. Ibuprofen and paracetamol for pain relief during medical abortion: A double-blind randomized controlled study. *Fertility and Sterility* 91(5):1877–1880.

Lohr, A. P., J. L. Hayes, and K. Gemzell Danielsson. 2008. Surgical versus medical methods for second trimester induced abortion. *Cochrane Database of Systematic Reviews* (1):CD006714.

Løkeland, M., O. E. Iversen, A. Engeland, I. Okland, and L. Bjorge. 2014. Medical abortion with mifepristone and home administration of misoprostol up to 63 days' gestation. *Acta Obstetricia et Gynecologica Scandinavica* 93(7):647–653.

Low, N., M. Mueller, H. A. Van Vliet, and N. Kapp. 2012. Perioperative antibiotics to prevent infection after first-trimester abortion. *Cochrane Database of Systematic Reviews* (3):CD005217.

Lydon-Rochelle M., V. L. Holt, T. R. Easterling, and D. P. Martin. 2001. Risk of uterine rupture during labor among women with a prior cesarean delivery. *New England Journal of Medicine* 345(1):3–8.

MacDorman, M. F., E. Declercq, and M. E. Thoma. 2017. Trends in maternal mortality by sociodemographic characteristics and cause of death in 27 states and the District of Columbia. *Obstetrics & Gynecology* 129(5):811–818.

Madden, T., J. L. Mullersman, K. J. Omvig, G. M. Secura, and J. F. Peipert. 2013. Structured contraceptive counseling provided by the Contraceptive CHOICE Project. *Contraception* 88(2):243–249.

Mark, K. S., B. Bragg, T. Talaie, K. Chawla, L. Murphy, and M. Terplan. 2017. Risk of complication during surgical abortion in obese women. *American Journal of Obstetrics and Gynecology* S0002-9378(17):31211–31215.

Mauelshagen, A., L. C. Sadler, H. Roberts, M. Harilall, and C. M. Farquhar. 2009. Audit of short term outcomes of surgical and medical second trimester termination of pregnancy. *Reproductive Health* 6(16):1–6.

McFarland, L. V. 1998. Epidemiology, risk factors and treatments for antibiotic-associated diarrhea. *Digestive Diseases* 16(5):292–307.

McNicholas, C., T. Madden, G. Secura, and J. F. Peipert. 2014. The Contraceptive CHOICE Project round up: What we did and what we learned. *Clinical Obstetrics and Gynecology* 57(4):635–643.

Meckstroth, K., and M. Paul. 2009. Chapter 5. First trimester aspiration abortion. In *Management of unintended and abnormal pregnancy: Comprehensive abortion care*, edited by M. Paul, E. S. Lichtenberg, L. Borgatta, D. A. Grimes, P. G. Stubblefield, and M. D. Creinin. Hoboken, NJ: Wiley-Blackwell. Pp. 135–156.

Moore, A. M., L. Frohwirth, and N. Blades. 2011. What women want from abortion counseling in the United States: A qualitative study of abortion patients in 2008. *Social Work in Health Care* 50(6):424–442.

Murphy, L. A., L. T. Thornburg, J. C. Glantz, E. C. Wasserman, N. L. Stanwood, and S. J. Betstadt. 2012. Complications of surgical termination of second-trimester pregnancy in obese versus nonobese women. *Contraception* 86(4):402–406.

NAF (National Abortion Federation). 2017a. *2017 Clinical policy guidelines for abortion care*. Washington, DC: NAF.

NAF. 2017b. *History*. https://prochoice.org/about-naf/history (accessed August 23, 2017).

Ngo, T. D., M. H. Park, H. Shakur, and C. Free. 2011. Comparative effectiveness, safety and acceptability of medical abortion at home and in a clinic: A systematic review. *Bulletin of the World Health Organisation* 89(5):360–370.

Ngoc, N. T., V. Q. Nhan, J. Blum, T. T. Mai, J. M. Durocher, and B. Winikoff. 2004. Is home-based administration of prostaglandin safe and feasible for medical abortion? Results from a multisite study in Vietnam. *BJOG: An International Journal of Obstetrics & Gynaecology* 111(8):814–819.

Ngoc, N. T., T. Shochet, S. Raghavan, J. Blum, N. T. Nga, N. T. Minh, V. Q. Phan, and B. Winikoff. 2011. Mifepristone and misoprostol compared with misoprostol alone for second-trimester abortion: A randomized controlled trial. *Obstetrics & Gynecology* 118(3):601–608.

Nichols, M., B. Halvofrson-Boyd, R. C. Goldstein, C. M. Gevirtz, and D. Healow. 2009. Chapter 8. Pain Management. In *Management of unintended and abnormal pregnancy: Comprehensive abortion care*, edited by M. Paul, E. S. Lichtenberg, L. Borgatta, D. A. Grimes, P. G. Stubblefield, and M. D. Creinin. Hoboken, NJ: Wiley-Blackwell. Pp. 90–110.

O'Connell, K., H. E. Jones, E. S. Lichtenberg, and M. Paul. 2008. Second-trimester surgical abortion practices: A survey of National Abortion Federation members. *Contraception* 78(6):492–499.

O'Connell, K., H. E. Jones, M. Simon, V. Saporta, M. Paul, and E. S. Lichtenberg. 2009. First-trimester surgical abortion practices: A survey of National Abortion Federation members. *Contraception* 79(5):385–392.

Ohannessian, A., K. Baumstarck, J. Maruani, E. Cohen-Solal, P. Auquier, and A. Agostini. 2016. Mifepristone and misoprostol for cervical ripening in surgical abortion between 12 and 14 weeks of gestation: A randomized controlled trial. *European Journal of Obstetrics & Gynecology and Reproductive Biology* 201:151–155.

Okusanya, B. O., O. Oduwole, and E. E. Effa. 2014. Immediate postabortal insertion of intrauterine devices. *Cochrane Database of Systematic Reviews* 28(7):CD0017777.

Patil, E., B. Darney, K. Orme-Evans, E. H. Beckley, L. Bergander, M. Nichols, P. H. Bednarek. 2016. Aspiration abortion with immediate intrauterine device insertion: Comparing outcomes of advanced practice clinicians and physicians. *Journal of Midwifery and Women's Health* 31(3):325–330.

Pazol, K., S. B. Gamble, W. Y. Parker, D. A. Cook, S. B. Zane, and S. Hamdan. 2009. Abortion surveillance—United States, 2006. *MMWR Surveillance Summaries* 58(8):1–35.

Peterson, W. F., F. N. Berry, M. R. Grace, and C. L. Gulbranson. 1983. Second-trimester abortion by dilatation and evacuation: An analysis of 11,747 cases. *Obstetrics & Gynecology* 62(2):185–190.

Platais, I., T. Tsereteli, G. Grebennikova, T. Lotarevich, and B. Winikoff. 2016. Prospective study of home use of mifepristone and misoprostol for medical abortion up to 10 weeks of pregnancy in Kazakhstan. *BJOG: An International Journal of Obstetrics & Gynaecology* 134(3):268–271.

Raymond, E. G., and D. A. Grimes. 2012. The comparative safety of legal induced abortion and childbirth in the United States. *Obstetrics and Gynecology* 119(2 Pt. 1):215–219.

Raymond, E. G., C. Shannon, M. A. Weaver, and B. Winikoff. 2013. First-trimester medical abortion with mifepristone 200 mg and misoprostol: A systematic review. *Contraception* 87(1):26–37.

Raymond, E. G., D. Grossman, M. A. Weaver, S. Toti, and B. Winikoff. 2014. Mortality of induced abortion, other outpatient surgical procedures and common activities in the United States. *Contraception* 90(5):476–479.

Raymond, E. G., D. Grossman, E. Wiebe, and B. Winikoff. 2015. Reaching women where they are: Eliminating the initial in-person medical abortion visit. *Contraception* 92(3):190–193.

Raymond, E. G., M. Weaver, K. S. Louie, Y. Tan, M. Bousiéguez, A. G. Aranguré-Peraza, E. M. Lugo-Hernández, P. Sanhueza, A. B. Goldberg, K. R. Culwell, C. Kaplan, L. Memmel, S. Sonalkar, R. Jamshidi, and B. Winikoff. 2016. Effect of depot medroxyprogesterone acetate injection timing on medical abortion efficacy and repeat pregnancy: A randomized controlled trial. *Obstetrics & Gynecology* 128(4):739–745.

RCOG (Royal College of Obstetricians and Gynaecologists). 2011. *The care of women requesting induced abortion* (Evidence-based clinical guideline number 7). https://www.rcog.org.uk/globalassets/documents/guidelines/abortion-guideline_web_1.pdf (accessed July 27, 2017).

RCOG. 2015. *Best practice in comprehensive abortion care* (Best practice paper no. 2). London, UK: RCOG.

RCOG. 2016. *Best practice in comprehensive postabortion care* (Best practice paper no. 3). London, UK: RCOG.

RCOG. 2017. *What we do.* https://www.rcog.org.uk/en/about-us/what-we-do (accessed August 23, 2017).

Renner, R. M., M. D. Nichols, J. T. Jensen, H. Li, and A. B. Edelman. 2012. Paracervical block for pain control in first-trimester surgical abortion: A randomized controlled trial. *Obstetrics and Gynecology* 119(5):1030–1037.

Renner, R. M., A. B. Edelman, M. D. Nichols, J. T. Jensen, J. Y. Lim, and P. H. Bednarek. 2016. Refining paracervical block techniques for pain control in first trimester surgical abortion: A randomized controlled noninferiority trial. *Contraception* 94(5):261–466.

Reumkens, A., E. J. Rondagh, C. M. Bakker, B. Winkens, A. A. Masclee, and S. Sanduleanu. 2016. Post-colonoscopy complications: A systematic review, time trends, and meta-analysis of population-based studies. *American Journal of Gastroenterology* 111(8):1092–1101.

RHN (Reproductive Health in Nursing). 2017. *Providing abortion care: A professional toolkit for nurse-midwives, nurse practitioners, and physician assistants.* https://rhnursing.org/resource/abortion-provider-toolkit-nurses (accessed October 20, 2017).

Roberts, S. C. 2017. *Research on facility-related factors and patient outcomes for non-hospital-based outpatient procedures.* Presentation to the Committee on Reproductive Health: Assessing the Safety and Quality of Abortion Care in the U.S. (Health and Medicine Division of the National Academies of Sciences, Engineering, and Medicine). Workshop on Facility Standards and the Safety of Outpatient Procedures, March 24, Washington, DC.

Roberts, S. C., H. Gould, K. Kimport, T. A. Weitz, and D. G. Foster. 2014. Out-of-pocket costs and insurance coverage for abortion in the United States. *Women's Health Issues* 24(2):e211–e218.

Roberts, S. C., D. K. Turok, E. Belusa, S. Combellick, and U. D. Upadhyay. 2016. Utah's 72-hour waiting period for abortion: Experiences among a clinic-based sample of women. *Perspectives on Sexual and Reproductive Health* 48(4):179–187.

Roblin, P. 2014. Vacuum aspiration. In *Abortion care,* edited by S. Rowlands. Cambridge, UK: Cambridge University Press. Pp. 71–79.

Rose, S. B., and B. A. Lawton. 2012. Impact of long-acting reversible contraception on return for repeat abortion. *American Journal of Obstetrics and Gynecology* 206(37):e1–e6.

Rosenstock, J. R., J. F. Peipert, T. Madden, Q. Zhao, and G. M. Secura. 2012. Continuation of reversible contraception in teenagers and young women. *Obstetrics & Gynecology* 120(6):1298–1305.

Russo, N. F., and J. E. Denious. 2001. Violence in the lives of women having abortions: Implications for practice and public policy. *Professional Psychology: Research and Practice* 32(2):142–150.

Sääv, I., O. Stephansson, and K. Gemzell-Danielsson. 2012. Early versus delayed insertion of intrauterine contraception after medical abortion—A randomized controlled trial. *PLoS One* 7(11):e48948.

Saftlas, A. F., A. B. Wallis, T. Shochet, K. K. Harland, P. Dickey, and C. Peek-Asa. 2010. Prevalence of intimate partner violence among an abortion clinic population. *American Journal of Public Health* 100(8):1412–1415.

Sanders, J. N., H. Conway, J. Jacobson, L. Torres, and D. K. Turok. 2016. The longest wait: Examining the impact of Utah's 72-hour waiting period for abortion. *Women's Health Issues* 26(5):483–487.

Secura, G. M., J. E. Allsworth, T. Madden, J. L. Mullersman, and J. F. Peipert. 2010. The Contraceptive CHOICE Project: Reducing barriers to long-acting reversible contraception. *American Journal of Obstetrics and Gynecology* 203(2):115.e1–115e.7.

SFP (Society for Family Planning). 2011a. Clinical guidelines. Labor induction abortion in the second trimester. *Contraception* 84(1):4–18.

SFP. 2011b. Prevention of infection after induced abortion. *Contraception* 83(4):295–309.

SFP. 2012. First-trimester abortion in women with medical conditions. *Contraception* 86(6):622–630.

SFP. 2013. Surgical abortion prior to 7 weeks of gestation. *Contraception* 88(1):7–17.

SFP. 2017. *Introducing SFP.* https://www.societyfp.org/About-SFP.aspx (accessed August 23, 2017).

Shannon, C. S., B. Winikoff, R. Hausknecht, E. Schaff, P. D. Blumenthal, D. Oyer, H. Sankey, J. Wolff, and R. Goldberg. 2005. Multicenter trial of a simplified mifepristone medical abortion regimen. *Obstetrics & Gynecology* 105(2):345–351.

Shrestha, A., and L. Sedhai. 2014. A randomized trial of hospital vs. home self administration of vaginal misoprostol for medical abortion. *Kathmandu University Medical Journal* 12(47):185–189.

Smalley, W. E., W. A. Ray, J. R. Daugherty, and M. R. Griffin. 1995. Nonsteroidal anti-inflammatory drugs and the incidence of hospitalizations for peptic ulcer disease in elderly persons. *American Journal of Epidemiology* 141(6):539–545.

Smith, R. L., N. Siddiqui, T. Henderson, J. Teresi, K. Downey, and J. C. Carvalho. 2016. Analgesia for medically induced second trimester termination of pregnancy: A randomized trial. *Journal of Obstetrics and Gynaecology Canada* 38(2):147–153.

Sonalkar, S., S. N. Ogden, L. K. Tran, and A. Y. Chen. 2017. Comparison of complications associated with induction by misoprostol versus dilation and evacuation for second-trimester abortion. *International Journal of Gynaecology & Obstetrics* 138(3):272–275.

Steinberg, J. R., and N. F. Russo. 2008. Abortion and anxiety: What's the relationship? *Social Science & Medicine* 67(2):238–252.

Strafford, M. A., J. Mottl-Santiago, A. Savla, N. Soodoo, and L. Borgatta. 2009. Relationship of obesity to outcome of medical abortion. *American Journal of Obstetrics and Gynecology* 200(5):e34–e36.

Swica, Y., E. Chong, T. Middleton, L. Prine, M. Gold, C. A. Schreiber, and B. Winikoff. 2013. Acceptability of home use of mifepristone for medical abortion. *Contraception* 88(1):122–127.

Taft, A. J., and Watson, L. F. 2007. Termination of pregnancy: Associations with partner violence and other factors in a national cohort of young Australian women. *Australian and New Zealand Journal of Public Health* 31(2):135–142.

Taft, A. J., L. F. Watson, and C. Lee. 2004. Violence against young Australian women and association with reproductive events: A cross-sectional analysis of a national population sample. *Australian and New Zealand Journal of Public Health* 28(4):324–329.

Tschann, M., J. Salcedo, and B. Kaneshiro. 2016. Nonpharmaceutical pain control adjuncts during first-trimester aspiration abortion: A review. *Journal of Midwifery & Women's Health* 61(3):331–338.

Upadhyay, U. D., T. A. Weitz, R. K. Jones, R. E. Barar, and D. G. Foster. 2014. Denial of abortion because of provider gestational age limits in the United States. *American Journal of Public Health* 104(9):1687–1694.

Upadhyay, U. D., S. Desai, V. Zlidar, T. A. Weitz, D. Grossman, P. Anderson, and D. Taylor. 2015. Incidence of emergency department visits and complications after abortion. *Obstetrics & Gynecology* 125(1):175–183.

Viviand, X., G. Fabre, D. Ortega, L. Boubli, and C. Martin. 2003. Target-controlled sedation analgesia using propofol and remifentanil in woman undergoing late termination of pregnancy. *International Journal of Obstetric Anesthesia* 12(2):83–88.

Whaley, N. S., and A. E. Burke. 2015. Update on medical abortion: Simplifying the process for women. *Current Opinion in Obstetrics and Gynecology* 27(6):476–481.

White, K., E. Carroll, and D. Grossman. 2015. Complications from first-trimester aspiration abortion: A systematic review of the literature. *Contraception* 92(5):422–438.

White, K., J. Turan, and D. Grossman. 2017. Travel for abortion services in Alabama and delays in obtaining care. *Women's Health Issues* 27(5):523–529.

WHO (World Health Organization). 2012. *Safe abortion: Technical and policy guidance for health systems*, 2nd ed. http://apps.who.int/iris/bitstream/10665/70914/1/9789241548434_eng.pdf (accessed September 12, 2017).

WHO. 2014. *Clinical practice handbook for safe abortion.* http://apps.who.int/iris/bitstream/10665/97415/1/9789241548717_eng.pdf?ua=1&ua=1 (accessed November 15, 2016).

WHO. 2015. *19th WHO model list of essential medicines (April 2015).* http://www.who.int/medicines/publications/essentialmedicines/EML2015_8-May-15.pdf (accessed March 10, 2017).

WHO. 2017. *About WHO.* http://www.who.int/about/what-we-do/en (accessed August 23, 2017).

Wiebe, E., and R. M. Renner. 2014. Chapter 11. Pain control. In *Abortion care*, edited by S. Rowlands. Cambridge, UK: Cambridge University Press. Pp. 98–105.

Wildschut, H., M. I. Both, S. Medema, E. Thomee, M. F. Wildhagen, and N. Kapp. 2011. Medical methods for mid-trimester termination of pregnancy. *Cochrane Database of Systematic Reviews* (1):CD005216.

Winner, B., J. F. Peipert, Q. Zhao, C. Buckel, T. Madden, J. E. Allsworth, and G. M. Secura. 2012. Effectiveness of long-acting reversible contraception. *New England Journal of Medicine* 366(21):1998–2007.

Woodcock, J. 2016. *Letter from the director of the FDA Center for Drug Evaluation and Research to Donna Harrison, Gene Rudd, and Penny Young Nance. Re: Docket No. FDA-2002-P-0364.* Silver Spring, MD: Food and Drug Administration.

Zane, S., A. A. Creanga, C. J. Berg, K. Pazol, D. B. Suchdev, D. J. Jamieson, and W. M. Callaghan. 2015. Abortion-related mortality in the United States: 1998–2010. *Obstetrics and Gynecology* 126(2):258–265.

Zurek, M., J. O'Donnell, R. Hart, and D. Rogow. 2015. Referral-making in the current landscape of abortion access. *Contraception* 91(1):1–5.

3

Essential Clinical Competencies
for Abortion Providers

Chapters 1 and 2 describe the elements of the continuum of abortion care services, including current abortion methods, relevant side effects and risks for complications, the appropriate clinical settings for the various abortion methods, state regulations affecting the quality of abortion care, and best practices for delivering high-quality, safe abortion care.

As part of its charge (see Box 1-1 in Chapter 1), the committee was tasked with reviewing the evidence on the clinical skills necessary for health care providers to safely perform the various components of abortion care, including pregnancy determination, counseling, gestation assessment, medication dispensing, procedure performance, patient monitoring, and follow-up assessment and care. Provider skills and training—significant factors that influence the safety and quality of abortion care—are the subject of this chapter.

Thus, this chapter identifies the clinical competencies for providing abortion care safely and with the highest degree of quality, the types of providers with the clinical competence to perform abortions, current abortion training of physicians and advanced practice clinicians (APCs), and the availability of appropriately trained clinicians. The chapter also describes the types of clinicians who provide abortion care in the United States; the available literature on the safety and quality of the care they provide; and current opportunities for education and training, including factors that affect the integration of abortion care in clinician education and training. A diverse range of providers can and do provide abortion care, although large-scale studies are generally limited to obstetrician/gynecologists (OB/GYNs), family medicine physicians, and APCs. This chapter focuses on these provider types because of the available data, but the committee recognizes that clinicians in other physician and health care specialties provide abortions and can be trained to provide safe and high-quality abortion care. This chapter also reviews abortion-specific state laws and policies that regulate the level of training and credentialing clinicians must have to be allowed to provide abortion services in different states. Finally, whereas this chapter focuses on provider skills and training, it is assumed the continuum of abortion care is being provided in a safe, well-organized setting/system of care and in an evidence-based manner, as described in Chapter 2.

REQUIRED CLINICAL COMPETENCIES

To determine the evidence-based, clinical competencies essential to providing high-quality abortion services, the committee reviewed clinical guidelines and training materials published by organizations that provide clinical guidance and continuing education to health professional students and clinicians. These sources include recommendations and standards issued by the American College of Obstetricians and Gynecologists (ACOG), Society of Family Planning (SFP), National Abortion Federation (NAF), Royal College of Obstetricians and Gynaecologists (RCOG), World Health Organization (WHO), University of California, San Francisco (UCSF) Bixby Center for Global Reproductive Health, Kenneth J. Ryan Residency Training Program, Fellowship in Family Planning, Reproductive Health Education in Family Medicine (RHEDI), Reproductive Health Access Project, and others.

For any clinical skill set, competency levels build on basic knowledge, didactic curriculum, clinical training, and continuing education. Key to the safety and quality of abortion services is having appropriate linkages in the continuum of care from preabortion services to postabortion services.

Some components of abortion care are consistent regardless of the particular abortion method; therefore, a number of essential competencies are required for any type of abortion procedure. These competencies have been outlined by several organizations, including the UCSF Bixby Center for Global Reproductive Health, NAF, the Fellowship in Family Planning, and the Ryan Residency Training Program, and include

- patient preparation (education, counseling, and informed consent);
- preprocedure assessment to confirm intrauterine pregnancy and assess gestation;
- pain management during and after the procedure;
- complication assessment and management; and
- provision of postabortion contraception and contraceptive counseling.

Additionally, the different abortion methods outlined in Chapter 2 (medication, aspiration, dilation and evacuation [D&E], and induction) require procedure-specific competencies. Increased gestation corresponds with increased procedural complexity; therefore, procedures performed later in pregnancy require more complex clinician competencies. See Table 3-1 for a list of all competencies by procedure type.

Patient Preparation

As noted in Chapter 2, patient preparation involves providing information to the patient about the available abortion methods (including pain

TABLE 3-1 Required Competencies by Type of Abortion Procedure

	Type of Procedure			
Competencies	Medication Abortion	Aspiration Abortion	Dilation and Evacuation (D&E)	Induction Abortion
Patient preparation (education, counseling, and informed consent)	√	√	√	√
Preprocedure evaluation	√	√	√	√
Complication assessment and management	√	√	√	√
Cervical preparation		√	√	√
Administration of abortion medications	√			√
Use of a manual or power vacuum extractor		√	√	
Forceps extraction			√	
Identification of products of conception		√	√	
Contraception provision	√	√	√	√
Pain management (techniques of analgesia and anesthesia)	√	√	√	√

SOURCES: ACOG, 2015; ACOG and SFP, 2014; Allen and Goldberg, 2016; Baird et al., 2007; Baker and Beresford, 2009; Creinin and Danielsson, 2009; Davis and Easterling, 2009; Goldstein and Reeves, 2009; Goodman et al., 2016; Hammond and Chasen, 2009; Kapp and von Hertzen, 2009; Meckstroth and Paul, 2009; NAF, 2017; Newmann et al., 2008, 2010; RCOG, 2015; SFP, 2014.

management options), the advantages and disadvantages of each method, potential side effects and risks for complications, and contraceptive options (ACOG and SFP, 2014; Goodman et al., 2016; NAF, 2017; Nichols et al., 2009; RCOG, 2015). For patients opting for sedation, a presedation evaluation is recommended (NAF, 2017). The patient's voluntary and informed consent for the procedure must also be obtained (Baker and Beresford, 2009; Goodman et al., 2016; NAF, 2017). During this process, the provider should provide accurate and understandable information and engage in shared decision making with the patient. Shared decision making is a process in which clinicians and patients work together to make decisions and select tests, treatments, and care plans based on clinical evidence that balances risks and expected outcomes with patient preferences and values (Health IT, 2013).

Preprocedure Assessment

A combination of diagnostic tests and physical examination can be used to confirm intrauterine pregnancy; assess gestation; screen for sexually transmitted infections (STIs) and cervical infections; document Rh status; and evaluate uterine size, position, anomalies, and pain (Goldstein and Reeves, 2009; Goodman et al., 2016; NAF, 2017; RCOG, 2015). Screening for anemia and evaluation for risk of bleeding are typically part of this preprocedure assessment and are often done by hemoglobin or hematocrit testing (NAF, 2017). Appropriate assessment also involves a medical history to determine relevant chronic or acute medical conditions, clinical risks, potential medication contraindications, and necessary modifications to care. Evaluation is necessary for developing a patient-centered clinical plan, determining the appropriate method and setting of abortion care, and knowing when to refer patients in need of more sophisticated clinical settings (Davis and Easterling, 2009; Goodman et al., 2016; RCOG, 2015).

Pain Management and Patient Support

Pain management varies based on patient preference, method of abortion, gestation, facility type, and availability of patient support from staff or others. Analgesia, anesthesia, and nonpharmacological pain management methods and risks are described in Chapter 2.

A member of the care team should discuss these options and risks with the patient during the patient preparation process, and if the patient opts for sedation, a presedation evaluation should be performed (Goodman et al., 2016; NAF, 2017; Nichols et al., 2009). A presedation evaluation includes relevant history and review of systems; medication review; targeted exam of the heart, lung, and airway; baseline vital signs; and last food intake (NAF, 2017). Providers must be able to administer paracervical blocks and nonsteroidal anti-inflammatory drugs to patients (NAF, 2017). If the patient opts for sedation or anesthesia, a supervising practitioner, appropriately trained to administer anesthesia and appropriately certified according to applicable local and state requirements, must be available (Goodman et al., 2016; NAF, 2017). To administer moderate sedation, NAF requires that a provider have appropriate licensure, basic airway skills, the ability to monitor and effectively rescue patients in an emergency, and the ability to screen patients appropriately (NAF, 2017). As noted above, providers must have the necessary resources and protocols for managing procedural and anesthesia complications and emergencies.

Procedure-related pain is a complex phenomenon influenced by multiple factors, including past history, anxiety, and individual tolerance. Relevant information about anticipated discomfort and options for pain management should be covered by the clinician during the informed consent process (Goodman et al., 2016; Nichols et al., 2009). The clinician should have a thorough understanding of potential side effects and complications from medications used to control pain.

Complication Assessment and Management

Assessment and management of abortion complications and medical emergencies are a key component of quality abortion care. Chapter 2 describes the types of complications that may require clinical follow-up. Although adverse events are rare, providers must have the ability to recognize conditions and risk factors associated with complications (e.g., accumulation of blood, retained tissue, excessive bleeding, and placental abnormalities) and have the resources or protocols necessary to manage these rare events. NAF and the UCSF Bixby Center recommend that providers have established protocols for medical emergencies, including bleeding and hemorrhage, perforation, respiratory arrest/depression, and anaphylaxis, and for emergency transfer (Goodman et al., 2016; NAF, 2017).

Contraception Provision and Counseling

Providing evidence-based information on how to prevent a future unintended pregnancy—including the option to obtain contraception contemporaneously with the procedure—is a standard component of abortion care (Goodman et al., 2016; NAF, 2017; RCOG, 2015; WHO, 2014). Contraceptive counseling should be patient-centered and guided by the patient's preferences (Goodman et al., 2016; RCOG, 2015). After the abortion, patients should receive the contraceptive method of their choice or be referred elsewhere if the preferred method is unavailable (NAF, 2017; RCOG, 2015; WHO, 2012). The Centers for Disease Control and Prevention and the U.S. Office of Population Affairs recommend the following for providers offering contraceptive services, including contraceptive counseling and education (Gavin et al., 2014):

- Establish and maintain rapport with the client.
- Obtain clinical and social information from the client (medical history, pregnancy intention, and contraceptive experiences and preferences).
- Work with the client interactively to select the most effective and appropriate contraceptive method (providers should ensure that patients understand the various methods' effectiveness, correct use, noncontraceptive benefits, side effects, and potential barriers to their use).
- Conduct a physical assessment related to contraceptive use, when warranted.
- Provide the selected contraceptive method along with instructions for its correct and consistent use, help the client develop a plan for using the selected method and for follow-up, and confirm the client's understanding of this information.

Competencies Required for Abortion Methods

Medication Abortion

Medication abortion is a method commonly used to terminate a pregnancy up to 70 days' (or 10 weeks') gestation with a combination of medications—mifepristone followed by misoprostol. The skill set required for early medication abortion has been outlined by several organizations and is similar to the management of spontaneous loss of a pregnancy with medications (Goodman et al., 2016). The skills include the essential competencies outlined in the section above, plus the knowledge of medication abortion protocols, associated health effects, and contraindications. Prescribing medication abortion is no different from prescribing other medications—providers must be able to recognize who is clinically eligible; counsel the patient regarding medication risks, benefits, and side effects; and instruct the patient on how to take the medication correctly and when to seek follow-up or emergency care.

Chapter 2 describes the U.S. Food and Drug Administration's (FDA's) Risk Evaluation and Mitigation Strategy (REMS) for Mifeprex, the brand name for mifepristone, the first drug administered during a medication abortion. Distribution of Mifeprex is restricted to REMS-certified health care providers, but any physician specialty or APC can become certified. In March 2016, the FDA issued revisions to the label and REMS for Mifeprex, changing the language from "physician" to "health care provider" and thereby expanding opportunities for APCs with relevant clinical competencies to obtain and distribute the drug (Simmonds et al., 2017; Woodcock, 2016). A component of the REMS process requires prescribers of Mifeprex to meet the following qualifications (FDA, 2016; Woodcock, 2016):

- ability to assess the duration of pregnancy accurately;
- ability to diagnose ectopic pregnancies; and
- ability to provide surgical intervention in cases of incomplete abortion or severe bleeding or have made plans to provide such care through others, and ability to ensure patient access to medical facilities equipped to provide blood transfusions and resuscitation, if necessary.

Aspiration Abortion

Aspiration abortion is a minimally invasive procedure that uses suction to empty the uterus. Aspiration abortion is an alternative to medication abortion up to 70 days' (or 10 weeks') gestation and the primary method of abortion through 13 weeks' gestation (Jatlaoui et al., 2016). The procedure and required skills are the same as those for the management of spontaneous loss of a pregnancy with uterine aspiration (Goodman et al., 2016; Nanda et al., 2012). The essential competencies for all abortion procedures form the basis of the skill set required for aspiration abortion. Additional competencies have been defined by the UCSF Bixby Center and NAF (Goodman et al., 2016; NAF, 2017). They include cervical preparation, experience with manual or electric vacuum aspiration, and evaluation of the products of conception for appropriate gestational tissue.

Dilation and Evacuation (D&E)

D&E is usually performed starting at 14 weeks' gestation, and most abortions after 14 weeks' gestation are performed by D&E (ACOG, 2015; Hammond and Chasen, 2009; Jatlaoui et al., 2016; O'Connell et al., 2008; Stubblefield et al., 2004). The procedure and required skills are similar to those for the surgical management of miscarriage after 14 weeks' gestation (Nanda et al., 2012). D&E requires clinicians with advanced training and/or experience, a more complex set of surgical skills relative to those required for aspiration abortion, and an adequate caseload to maintain these surgical skills (Gemzell-Danielsson and Lalitkumar, 2008;

Grossman et al., 2008; Hammond and Chasen, 2009; Hern, 2016; Kapp and von Hertzen, 2009; Lohr et al., 2008; RCOG, 2015). The additional skills required for D&E include surgical expertise in D&E provision and training in the use of specialized forceps. Cervical preparation, achieved by osmotic dilators or prostaglandin analogues (misoprostol), is standard practice for D&E after 14 weeks' gestation (Newmann et al., 2008, 2010; SFP, 2014).

Induction Abortion

Induction abortion is the termination of pregnancy using medications to induce delivery of the fetus. Induction abortion requires a clinician skilled in cervical preparation and delivery (ACOG, 2015; Baird et al., 2007; Hammond and Chasen, 2009; Kapp and von Hertzen, 2009). As with any woman in labor, providing supportive care for women undergoing induction abortion is of utmost importance. Physical as well as emotional support should be offered (Baird et al., 2007). Women should be encouraged to have a support person with them if possible.

WHICH PROVIDERS HAVE THE CLINICAL SKILLS TO PERFORM ABORTIONS?

While OB/GYNs provide the greatest percentage of abortions (O'Connell et al., 2008, 2009), other types of clinicians (both generalist physicians and APCs) also perform abortions. The committee identified systematic reviews, randomized controlled trials, and a variety of cohort studies assessing the outcomes of abortions provided by family medicine physicians or comparing the outcomes of abortions performed by physicians and nurse practitioners (NPs), certified nurse-midwives (CNMs), and/or physician assistants (PAs) (Bennett et al., 2009; Goldman et al., 2004; Kopp Kallner et al., 2015; Ngo et al., 2013; Paul et al., 2007; Prine et al., 2010; Renner et al., 2013; Weitz et al., 2013). Many of the comparative studies were based in parts of the world where provider shortages are particularly acute, often in developing countries. All the available systematic reviews include this international research and also judge much of the research to be of poor quality (Barnard et al., 2015; Ngo et al., 2013; Renner et al., 2013; Sjöström et al., 2017). The literature is less robust regarding other generalist physicians, yet the same judgment and clinical dexterity necessary to perform first-trimester abortion are possessed by many specialties.

This section reviews the primary research on which providers have the clinical skills to provide abortions that is most relevant to the delivery of abortion care in the United States. It is noteworthy that numerous professional and health care organizations, including ACOG, NAF, the American

Public Health Association, WHO, and others,[1] endorse APCs providing abortion care (ACOG, 2014a,b; APHA, 2011; Goodman et al., 2016; NAF, 2017; WHO, 2014, 2015).

Medication and Aspiration Abortion

Advanced Practice Clinicians

The committee identified three primary research studies that assessed APCs' skills in providing either medication or aspiration abortions.

The Health Workforce Pilot Project (HWPP) was a 6-year multisite prospective clinical competency-based training program and study sponsored by the Advancing New Standards in Reproductive Health (ANSIRH) program at the UCSF Bixby Center. The project was designed to train APCs to competence in the provision of aspiration abortion and to evaluate the safety, effectiveness, and acceptability of APCs providing abortion care, in an effort to expand the number of trained providers in California (ANSIRH, 2014; Levi et al., 2012; Weitz et al., 2013). The project received a waiver from the California Office of Statewide Health Planning and Development (OSHPD) to proceed with the study because of an existing statute that limited the provision of aspiration abortion to physicians (Weitz et al., 2013). The project used the Training in Early Abortion for Comprehensive Healthcare model, which combines didactic learning, clinical skill development, and a variety of evaluation methods to ensure clinical competency (Levi et al., 2012).

Weitz and colleagues (2013) evaluated the patient outcomes of aspiration abortions provided between August 2007 and August 2011 by physicians and APCs from five partner organizations, trained to competence through HWPP. The analysis included 11,487 aspiration abortions performed by 40 APCs (n = 5,675) and 96 OB/GYN or family medicine physicians (n = 5,812). The complication rate was 1.8 percent for APCs and 0.9 percent for physicians, with no clinically relevant margin of difference (95% confidence interval [CI] = 1.11, 1.53) (Weitz et al., 2013). The authors concluded that APCs can be trained to competence in early abortion care and provide safe abortion care.

The patients in the study (n = 9,087) completed a survey after their abortions to enable the investigators to assess the women's experience,

---

[1]The American Academy of Physician Assistants, the American College of Nurse-Midwives, the American Medical Women's Association, the Association of Physician Assistants in Obstetrics and Gynecology, the International Confederation of Midwives, the National Association of Nurse Practitioners in Women's Health, and Physicians for Reproductive Choice and Health also support an increased role for appropriately trained APCs (ACNM, 2011b; ICM, 2011b; NAF and CFC, 2018).

access to care, and health; regardless of clinician type, the patient experience scores were very high (Taylor et al., 2013). Treatment by staff, timeliness of care, and level of pain were factors that highly impacted women's rating of their experience, but patient experience was not statistically different by clinician type after controlling for other patient- and clinic-level factors.

A qualitative analysis of the women's responses to the survey's open-ended question on their experience (n = 5,214) was conducted to determine themes across the responses (McLemore et al., 2014). The responses were categorized into themes of factors at the patient level (experiences of shame/stigma, pain experience, and interactions with staff) and clinic level (perceptions of clinical environment, adequate pain management, and wait time). Almost 97 percent of respondents reported their patient experience to be what they had expected or better. Major themes identified in the responses by women who reported their experience to have been worse than expected included issues with clinical care (problems with intravenous line insertion and/or preprocedure ultrasound, uncertainty about abortion completion, and needing subsequent follow-up appointments), level of pain experienced, and frustration with wait times for appointments and within the clinic.

In summary, the HWPP studies found that aspiration abortions were performed safely and effectively by both APCs and physicians and with a high degree of patient satisfaction (McLemore et al., 2014; Taylor et al., 2013; Weitz et al., 2013). The project, overseen by OSHPD, was completed in 2013, and the study results supported new legislation[2] in California that expanded the scope of practice for APCs to include early abortion care.

Two smaller studies compared the outcomes of abortions performed by APCs and physicians. In a 2-year prospective cohort study, Goldman and colleagues (2004) analyzed the outcomes of aspiration abortions provided by three PAs in a Vermont clinic (n = 546) and three physicians (n = 817) in a New Hampshire clinic. The authors found no statistically significant difference[3] in the complication rates of the two types of clinicians. Kopp Kallner and colleagues (2015) conducted a nonblinded randomized equivalence trial comparing medication abortions (using the WHO protocol and routine ultrasound) performed by 2 nurse-midwives and 34 physicians in Sweden. The primary outcome was defined as successful completion of the abortion without the need for a follow-up aspiration procedure. Complication rates and women's views on the acceptability of nonphysician providers were also assessed. The results showed superiority for the nurse-midwife group. The risk ratio for the physician group was 2.5 (95% CI =

---

[2]California Assembly Bill No. 154 to amend California Business and Professions Code, Section 2253 and California Health and Safety Code, Section 123468.
[3]The threshold for statistical significance was $p \leq .05$.

1.4, 4.3). The researchers concluded that using nurse-midwives to provide early medication abortions is highly effective in high-resource areas such as theirs.

Family Medicine Physicians

Multiple studies have concluded that family medicine physicians provide medication and aspiration abortions safely and effectively (Bennett et al., 2009; Paul et al., 2007; Prine et al., 2003, 2010) with a high degree of patient satisfaction (Paul et al., 2007; Prine et al., 2010; Summit et al., 2016; Wu et al., 2015). In one study of 2,550 women who sought abortions in five clinical settings from family physicians, medication and aspiration procedures had a 96.5 percent and 99.1 percent success rate, respectively (Bennett et al., 2009). All complications were minor and managed effectively at rates similar to those in OB/GYN practices and specialty abortion clinics. Another study of 847 medication abortions in a family medicine setting similarly found that the abortions were as safe and effective as those provided in specialty clinics (Prine et al., 2010).

The literature is less robust regarding other generalist physicians. However, the same judgment and clinical dexterity necessary to perform medication and aspiration abortions are obtained in other specialty training.

D&E and Induction Abortions

The committee could identify no comparative studies of clinicians who perform D&E and induction abortions. In the United States, D&Es are performed by OB/GYNs, family medicine physicians, or other physicians with advanced training and/or experience (such as the training provided in specialized fellowships) (O'Connell et al., 2008; Steinauer et al., 2012). In general, OB/GYNs have the most experience in the surgical techniques used to perform a D&E abortion. Induction abortion can be provided by a team of providers with the requisite skill set for managing women in labor and during delivery, such as OB/GYNs, family medicine physicians, and CNMs (Gemzell-Danielsson and Lalitkumar, 2008).

TRAINING OF PHYSICIANS AND ADVANCED PRACTICE CLINICIANS

Although most women's health care providers will interact with patients navigating issues of unintended pregnancy and abortion, abortion training is not universally available to physicians or APCs who intend to provide reproductive health services. Evidence suggests that few education programs incorporate abortion training in didactic curriculum, and only a small percentage of residencies, regardless of type or specialty, with the exception of OB/GYN, offer integrated abortion training (Herbitter et al., 2011, 2013; Lesnewski et al., 2003; Steinauer et al., 1997; Talley and Bergus, 1996; Turk et al., 2014).

Many factors influence the availability of training, including geography, institutional policy, and state law. Additionally, training has become more limited as a result of religious hospital mergers, state restrictions on medical schools and hospitals used for training programs, and training inconsistencies (Goodman et al., 2016). Catholic and Catholic-owned health care institutions are the largest group of religiously owned nonprofit hospitals, governing 15 percent of all acute care hospitals and 17 percent of hospital beds in the United States, and in many areas, these institutions function as the sole community hospital.[4] Employees at these institutions are bound by *Ethical and Religious Directives for Catholic Health Care Services*, which prohibits providing and teaching certain reproductive services, including abortion (Freedman and Stulberg, 2013; Freedman et al., 2008; Stulberg et al., 2016). Medical students, residents, and other health professional students are often responsible for seeking out learning opportunities themselves, as almost all abortions are provided outside of the traditional health care trainee learning environment (ACOG, 2014a,b).

Obstetrics and Gynecology

The organization that accredits allopathic (and by 2020, also osteopathic) residencies in the United States is the Accreditation Council for Graduate Medical Education (ACGME). The ACGME training requirements for OB/GYN state that (1) programs must provide training or access to training in the provision of abortions, and this must be part of a planned curriculum; (2) residents who have religious or moral objections may opt out and must not be required to participate; and (3) residents must have experience in managing complications of abortions and training in all forms of contraception, including reversible methods and sterilization (ACGME, 2017b). Although this requirement has been in place since 1996, a number of OB/GYN residency programs do not provide specific training in abortion, and others provide such training only at the request of the resident (opt-in training). In 1995, Congress passed the Coates Amendment of the Omnibus Consolidated Rescissions and Appropriations Act of 1996,[5] which upholds the legal status and federal funding of institutions that do

---

[4]Designated by the Centers for Medicare & Medicaid Services if the hospital is at least 35 miles from other like hospitals or if travel time between the hospital and the nearest like hospital is at least 45 minutes.

[5]S971, 104th Congress, 1st session (1995).

not provide abortion training or referrals for residents seeking such training elsewhere (Tocce and Severson, 2012). While the federal funding to these institutions may be preserved, this legislation does not shield institutional residency programs from the need to comply with the accreditation requirements put forth by ACGME.

Although the majority of abortion providers are OB/GYNs (O'Connell et al., 2008, 2009), available data indicate that most OB/GYNs do not provide abortions. Stulberg and colleagues (2011) surveyed practicing OB/GYNs in 2008–2009 using the American Medical Association Physician Masterfile to determine the extent to which OB/GYNs were providing abortions. Of the 1,144 respondents, 14.4 percent provided abortions, whereas 97 percent reported encountering an abortion-seeking patient. OB/GYNs located in the Northeastern or Western United States and those whose zip code was greater than 90 percent urban were most likely to provide abortions (Stulberg et al., 2011). According to the most recent data collected from NAF members, approximately 64 percent of NAF member providers who performed first-trimester surgical abortions in 2001 were OB/GYNs (O'Connell et al., 2009). These are the most recent data available for NAF members, but given the growing percentage of medication abortions before 10 weeks' gestation and expanded opportunities for other types of providers, APCs and family physicians may now represent an increased share of abortion providers.

A 2014 study of OB/GYN fourth-year residents associated with 161 of the 248 total residency programs found that 54 percent of residents reported routine abortion training; 30 percent reported opt-in training, where the training was available but not integrated; and 16 percent reported that training in elective abortion was unavailable in their program (Turk et al., 2014). Previous studies have found training participation rates to be very low among programs with optional training (Almeling et al., 2000; Eastwood et al., 2006).

From their general training, OB/GYN physicians may be more experienced with the surgical techniques of D&E and dilation and sharp curettage (D&C) relative to medication abortion (ACOG, 2015). In a 2007 survey of OB/GYNs who had recently completed their residencies, 65.1 percent reported receiving training in D&C, 62.0 percent in D&E, and 60.2 percent in induction. Residents had received the least training in medication abortion—40.7 percent reported training in mifepristone and misoprostol provision, 43.5 percent in manual vacuum aspiration (MVA), and 45.1 percent in electric vacuum aspiration. Thus, the residents had received more training in abortion procedures that are performed after 13 weeks' gestation. Of the 324 respondents, 62 percent indicated that it was easy to not participate in abortion training (Jackson and Foster, 2012).

Kenneth J. Ryan Residency Training Program

The Ryan Program, developed by the UCSF Bixby Center in 1999, aims to integrate and enhance family planning training for OB/GYN residents in the United States and Canada (Ryan Residency Training Program, 2017a). The program offers resources and technical expertise to OB/GYN departments that wish to establish a formal, opt-out rotation in family planning (Ryan Residency Training Program, 2017a). Among the total 269 accredited OB/GYN residency programs across the United States during the 2016–2017 academic year, there are 90 Ryan programs[6] (see Figure 3-1), and as of December 2016, 3,963 residents had graduated from Ryan programs (ACGME, 2017c; Ryan Residency Training Program, 2017b).

The Ryan curriculum consists of published comprehensive didactic learning modules and expected milestones for all aspects of abortion care, including contraceptive counseling (Ryan Residency Training Program, 2017c). These milestones distinguish among the necessary clinical competencies for residents-in-training, graduating residents, and area experts. Graduating residents must independently perform procedures (first-trimester aspiration and basic second-trimester D&E) and manage medication abortions and labor induction terminations; manage complications of the different types of abortion procedures; and determine the need for consultation, referral, or transfer of patients with complex conditions, such as those with medical comorbidities or prior uterine surgery.

In annual reviews of the Ryan Program, residents and program directors have reported significant exposure to all methods of abortion and contraception provision, as well as such broader gynecological skills as anesthesia and analgesia, uterine sizing, assessment of gestation, ultrasound, management of fetal demise, and management of abortion-related complications (Steinauer et al., 2013b). In a study by Steinauer and colleagues (2013a), most residents and program directors reported believing that both full and partial program participation improved residents' knowledge and skills in counseling, contraception provision, and uterine evacuation for indications other than elective abortion, such as therapeutic abortion, miscarriage, and suspected ectopic management.

Fellowship in Family Planning

Other training opportunities include the Fellowship in Family Planning, a 2-year postresidency fellowship program that offers comprehensive training in research, teaching, and clinical practice in abortion and contraception

---

[6]Personal communication, U. Landy, Ph.D., UCSF Bixby Center for Global Reproductive Health, March 30, 2017.

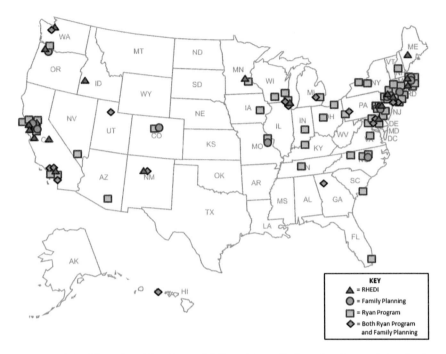

FIGURE 3-1 Selected residencies and fellowships offering abortion training in the United States.
NOTE: RHEDI = Reproductive Health Education in Family Medicine.
SOURCES: FFP, 2017; RHEDI, 2017; Ryan Residency Training Program, 2017b.

at academic medical centers. The fellowship is offered at 30 university locations (see Figure 3-1) and is available to OB/GYNs who have completed residency training (FFP, 2017). Currently, 64 fellows are enrolled in these 2-year programs, and 275 physicians have completed the fellowship training (FFP, 2017).

Family Medicine

Women's reproductive health care is a fundamental component of family medicine. Family physicians provide routine gynecological, pregnancy counseling, obstetrics, and contraceptive services (Brahmi et al., 2007; Dehlendorf et al., 2007; Goodman et al., 2013; Herbitter et al., 2011; Rubin et al., 2011). ACGME requires that family medicine trainees have 100 hours (or 1 month) or 125 patient encounters in gynecological care, including family planning, miscarriage management, contraceptive services, and options counseling for unintended pregnancy (ACGME, 2017a). The

Society of Teachers of Family Medicine (STFM) Group on Hospital and Procedural Training recommends that all family medicine residents be exposed to uterine aspirations and D&Cs and have the opportunity to train to independent performance as these procedures are used for a variety of gynecological conditions (Nothnagle et al., 2008). Thus, although there is no specific abortion training requirement in family medicine, residents learn many gynecological skills that are applicable to performing abortions (e.g., counseling, aspirations, endometrial biopsies, and intrauterine device insertion and removal) (AAFP, 2016; Lyus et al., 2009). Indeed, the American Academy of Family Physicians considers medication and aspiration abortions to be within the scope of family medicine (AAFP, 2016).

Available data indicate that most family physicians do not provide abortions. A 2012 survey of 1,198 responding academic family medicine physicians found that only 15.3 percent of respondents had ever provided an abortion (medical or surgical) outside of training, and of those, only 33.8 percent had performed an abortion in the previous year (Herbitter et al., 2013). According to the most recent data collected from NAF members, 21 percent of NAF member providers who performed aspiration abortions in 2001 specialized in family practice (O'Connell et al., 2009). The 2016 National Graduate Survey, conducted by the American Board of Family Medicine and the Association of Family Medicine Residency Directors, was administered to 2013 graduates of residency training. When asked about specific subject areas and procedures, 17 percent of respondents (n = 2,060) reported that residency had prepared them in uterine aspiration/D&C, and 4 percent of respondents (n = 2,034) reported currently practicing these procedures.[7]

Most family medicine programs do not offer specific training in abortion, and only a small proportion of family physicians report having had access to abortion training (Herbitter et al., 2011, 2013; Lesnewski et al., 2003; Steinauer et al., 1997; Talley and Bergus, 1996). In a 2007–2008 survey of family medicine chief residents and program directors, almost two-thirds (63.9 percent) of residents reported that training in medication and aspiration abortions was not available in their programs (Herbitter et al., 2011).

The total number of family medicine residencies offering abortion training is unknown, although it is clear that access to such training varies markedly across the country (Herbitter et al., 2011; Steinauer et al., 1997; Talley et al., 1996). Programs in the West and Northeast are far more likely to provide abortion training relative to programs in the Midwest and South (Herbitter et al., 2011). In 2002, the STFM Group on Abortion Training

---

[7]Personal communication, L. Peterson, M.D., Ph.D., American Board of Family Medicine, January 30, 2018.

and Access conducted a survey of family medicine residency programs to determine the levels of abortion training offered. They confirmed that only 3.3 percent (11 of 337) of responding programs offered fully integrated abortion training (Lesnewski et al., 2003). In programs where abortion training is available, it appears that curricula are quite variable. A 2004–2005 study of nine programs that required abortion training found that all nine provided training in vacuum aspiration, eight of the nine provided training in medication abortion, and eight of the nine offered ultrasound training (Brahmi et al., 2007). The clinical setting, duration, and content of nonprocedural training were not consistent across the nine programs (Brahmi et al., 2007).

In addition to the RHEDI programs discussed below, seven family medicine residency programs offer integrated and comprehensive abortion training, and two programs offer established local electives in abortion training (RHEDI, 2017) (see Figure 3-1).

RHEDI

The RHEDI program includes 26 family medicine residency programs with fully integrated abortion and family planning training—5.2 percent of the total 498 accredited family medicine residency programs in 2016 (ACGME, 2016; RHEDI, 2017; Summit and Gold, 2017) (see Figure 3-1). RHEDI, established in 2004 at the Montefiore Medical Center, provides grant funding and technical assistance to establish RHEDI programs in family medicine residencies throughout the United States. In a 2012–2014 evaluation of 214 residents in 12 RHEDI programs (representing 90 percent of residents who were part of a RHEDI program during the time period), residents reported increased exposure to provision of contraception (all methods), counseling on pregnancy options, counseling on abortion methods, ultrasound, aspiration and medication abortions, and miscarriage management after their RHEDI rotation. Self-rated competency had also improved (Summit and Gold, 2017). RHEDI is in the process of developing a standardized curriculum.[8]

Fellowship in Family Planning

The previously mentioned Fellowships in Family Planning are available to family physicians that have completed residency training. Three of the 30 fellowship sites (see Figure 3-1) are housed in departments of family

---

[8]Personal communication, M. Gold, M.D., Albert Einstein College of Medicine, June 27, 2017.

medicine (FFP, 2017). Additionally, 2 of the 84 Ryan Residency Training programs are available to family physicians.[9]

Advanced Practice Clinicians

State licensing boards govern the scope of practice for APCs. CNMs and NPs are first credentialed as registered nurses and then as advanced practice nurses in a CNM or NP role. APCs may be educated and also credentialed to practice with a specific population (e.g., primary care, women's health) and/or a specialty area (e.g., abortion care) (Taylor et al., 2009).

Professional regulation and credentialing are based on a set of essential elements that align government authority with regulatory and professional responsibilities. The latter include essential documents developed by the profession that provide a basis for education and practice regulation; formal education from a degree or professional certification program; formal accreditation of educational programs; legal scope of practice by state law and regulations, including licensure; and individual certification formally recognizing the knowledge, skills, and experience of the individual to meet the standards the profession has identified (Taylor et al., 2009).

Foster and colleagues (2006) conducted a survey of all 486 accredited NP, PA, and CNM programs in the United States, with a response rate of 42 percent (n = 202). Overall, 53 percent of responding programs (108 programs) reported didactic instruction in surgical abortion,[10] MVA, and/or medication abortion; 21 percent (43 programs) reported providing clinical instruction in at least one of the three abortion procedures (Foster et al., 2006).

Abortion care competencies are operationalized within individual APC educational programs. In the Foster et al. (2006) study, among all APC educational programs, accredited CNM programs reported the highest rates of didactic instruction in abortion, and accredited NP programs reported the lowest rates of didactic and clinical instruction. Training in abortion care is very difficult for APCs to access. Planned Parenthood Federation of America's Consortium of Abortion Providers offers some training to the federation's members. NAF offers some didactic and practicum training in abortion care, as well as accredited continuing medical education, that is available to APCs (Taylor et al., 2009). Additionally, the Midwest Access Project (MAP) provides connection to training sites for APCs, although MDs receive priority in its placements (MAP, 2017).

---

[9]Personal communication, U. Landy, Ph.D., UCSF Bixby Center for Global Reproductive Health, March 30, 2017.

[10]The authors note a preference for the term "electric vacuum aspiration" to clarify "surgical abortion" in future surveys.

Certified Nurse-Midwives (CNMs)

Midwifery practice encompasses the full range of women's primary care services, including primary care; family planning; STI treatment; gynecological services; care during pregnancy, childbirth, and postpartum; and newborn care (ACNM, 2011a).

CNMs are prepared at the graduate level in educational programs accredited by the Accreditation Commission for Midwifery Education, and must pass a national certification examination administered by the American Midwifery Certification Board. The competencies and standards for the practice of midwifery in the United States are consistent with or exceed the global competencies and standards set forth by the International Confederation of Midwives, including, for example, uterine evacuation via MVA (ICM, 2011a, 2013). These competencies are outlined in *Core Competencies for Basic Midwifery Practice* and must be met by an individual graduating from an accredited midwifery program (ACNM, 2012).

While abortion care is not specifically identified as a core competency for basic midwifery practice, CNMs have the essential skills to be trained to provide medication and aspiration abortions. The scope of midwifery practice may be expanded beyond the core competencies to incorporate additional skills and procedures, such as aspiration abortion, by following the guidelines outlined in Standard VIII of *Standards for the Practice of Midwifery* (ACNM, 2011c).

Nurse Practitioners (NPs)

NPs receive advanced education (typically a master's degree or clinical doctorate) and extensive clinical training to enable them to diagnose and manage patient care for a multitude of acute and chronic illnesses. They are independently licensed, have prescriptive authority in some form in all states, and work collaboratively with other health care professionals (Taylor et al., 2009). Their competencies are outlined in *Nurse Practitioner Core Competencies*, issued by the National Organization of Nurse Practitioner Faculties (NONPF, 2017).

The *Consensus Model for APRN Regulation* provides for the expansion of all NP and nurse-midwifery practice roles to advance their practice beyond the core competencies, providing flexibility to meet the emerging and changing needs of patients (APRN and NCSBN, 2008). Competency can be acquired through practical, supervised experience or through additional education and assessed in multiple ways through professional credentialing mechanisms.

Physician Assistants (PAs)

PA training programs are accredited by the Accreditation Review Commission on Education for the Physician Assistant (ARC-PA). There is no mandated specific curriculum for PA schools, nor is there mandated abortion or family planning training for PAs. The ARC-PA Practice Standards include supervised clinical training in women's health (to include prenatal and gynecological care) (ARC-PA, 2010). The National Commission on Certification of Physician Assistants prepares and administers certifying and recertifying examinations for PAs. The 2015 Content Blueprint includes abortion in its list of reproductive system diseases for the examinations. The Association of Physician Assistants in Obstetrics & Gynecology (APAOG) highlights two OB/GYN residencies, but these residencies do not offer specific abortion training, and most PAs are trained privately in abortion procedures by supervising physicians at their practice sites (APAOG, 2017).

Expansion of the scope of practice for PAs varies slightly from that for advanced practice nurses. Most state laws governing the scope of practice for PAs allow for broad delegatory authority by the supervising physician. The American Academy of Physician Assistants (AAPA) recommends that all PAs consider four parameters when incorporating new skills into their practice: state law, facility policies, delegatory decisions made by the supervising physician, and the PA's education and experience (AAPA, 2017).

AVAILABILITY OF TRAINED CLINICIANS

The safety and quality of abortion services are contingent on the availability of skilled providers. A number of issues influence the availability of providers skilled in abortion services, including the declining number of facilities offering services (discussed in Chapter 1), the geographic maldistribution of providers, and legal restrictions on training in and provision of services.

Geographic Distribution

There are marked geographic disparities in a woman's ability to access abortion services in the United States, mirroring the locations of fellowship and residency programs in family planning. Abortion providers tend to be concentrated in urban areas, and a paucity of abortion providers exists in the South and Midwest, creating geographic barriers for women seeking abortion services in these regions (Johns et al., 2017; Jones and Jerman, 2017a; Paul and Norton, 2016). In 2011, 53 percent of women in the Midwest and 49 percent of women in the South lived in a county without an abortion clinic, compared with 24 percent of women in the Northeast and 16 percent of women in the West (Jones and Jerman, 2014). In 2008, women traveled an average of 30 miles for an abortion, with 17 percent traveling more than 50 miles (Jones and Jerman, 2013). Among women living in rural areas, 31 percent traveled more than 100 miles to have an abortion (Jones and Jerman, 2013).

A significant amount of qualitative and quantitative research has been conducted to evaluate the impact of a 2013 law (H.B. 2)[11] that resulted in a reduced number of abortion facilities in Texas. The law went into effect in November 2013, and the number of Texas clinics subsequently declined from 41 in May 2013 to 17 in June 2016 (Grossman et al., 2014, 2017).

Researchers compared the 6-month periods before and after the implementation of the law and found that in the 6 months after implementation, the abortion rate decreased by 13 percent, the proportion of abortions at or after 12 weeks' gestation increased, and medication abortion decreased by 70 percent (Grossman et al., 2014). Furthermore, women had to travel an increased distance for abortion care. The number of women of reproductive age living more than 200 miles from an abortion facility increased from approximately 10,000 in the 6 months prior to the law's implementation to 290,000 6 months after implementation. The number of women living more than 50 and 100 miles from a facility increased from approximately 800,000 to 1.7 million and 400,000 to nearly 1.1 million, respectively (Grossman et al., 2014). Gerdts and colleagues (2016) surveyed women seeking abortion care in 2014 and found that those whose nearest clinic closed in 2013 traveled on average 85 miles to obtain care, compared with 22 miles traveled by women whose nearest clinic remained open. A later study by Grossman and colleagues (2017) found that the decline in abortions increased as the distance to the nearest facility increased between 2012 and 2014. Counties with no change in distance to a facility saw a 1.3 percent decline in abortions, whereas counties with an increase in distance of 100 miles or more saw a 50.3 percent decline (Grossman et al., 2017). Women reported increased informational, cost, and logistical barriers to obtaining abortion services; increased cost and travel time; and a frustrated demand for medication abortion after the law took effect (Baum et al., 2016; Fuentes et al., 2016; Gerdts et al., 2016).

Geographic location figures prominently in equitable access to abortion providers, impacting both the quality and safety of abortion care for women. A 2011–2012 study of claims data on 39,747 abortions covered by California's state Medicaid program (named Medi-Cal) found that

---

[11]Texas House Bill 2 (Tex. Health & Safety Code Ann. § 171.0031[a] [West Cum. Supp. 2015]) banned abortions after 20 weeks postfertilization, required physicians performing abortions to have hospital admitting privileges within 30 miles of the abortion facility, required the provision of medication abortion to follow the labeling approved by the FDA, and required all abortion facilities to be ambulatory surgery centers (Grossman et al., 2014).

12 percent of the women traveled 50 miles or more for abortion services, and 4 percent traveled more than 100 miles (Upadhyay et al., 2017). For most patients in this study, greater distance traveled was associated with an increased likelihood of seeking follow-up care at a local emergency department, driving up cost and interrupting continuity of care. Women traveling longer distances (25–49 miles, 50–99 miles, or 100 miles or more) were significantly more likely than those traveling 25 miles or less to seek follow-up care in a local emergency department instead of returning to their original provider (Upadhyay et al., 2017). Costs associated with emergency department care were consistently higher than those of follow-up care at the abortion site. In addition to disrupting continuity of care and increasing medical costs, emergency department visits are not the ideal avenue for follow-up abortion care. Evidence suggests that abortion providers are better prepared than emergency department staff to evaluate women post-abortion, avoiding unnecessary use of such interventions as repeat aspiration or antibiotics (Beckman et al., 2002). This finding suggests a disparity in quality of abortion care for women unable to return to their abortion site for follow-up.

As demonstrated in Texas after passage of H.B. 2, geographic disparities contribute to increased travel and logistic challenges for women seeking abortion care, which in turn can result in delays (Bessett et al., 2011; Drey et al., 2006; Finer et al., 2006; Foster and Kimport, 2013; French et al., 2016; Fuentes et al., 2016; Janiak et al., 2014; Kiley et al., 2010; Roberts et al., 2014; Upadhyay et al., 2014; White et al., 2016). Restrictive regulations, including mandatory waiting periods that require a woman to make multiple trips to the abortion facility, impact the timeliness of obtaining abortion care (Grossman et al., 2014; Jones and Jerman, 2016). These challenges are especially burdensome for poor women, women traveling long distances for care, and those with the fewest resources (Baum et al., 2016; Finer et al., 2006; Fuentes et al., 2016; Ostrach and Cheyney, 2014). Delays in obtaining care may result in later abortions, requiring procedures with greater clinical risks and increased costs, in addition to limiting patient options regarding abortion procedures and pain management.

As noted in Chapter 1, most women pay out of pocket for abortions (Jones and Jerman, 2017b). A 2012 survey of nonhospital abortion facilities estimated that at 10 weeks' gestation, the average charge for an aspiration abortion was $480 and for a medication abortion was $504 (Jerman and Jones, 2014). The median charge for an abortion at 20 weeks' gestation was $1,350.

The availability of providers also varies by gestation. Far fewer clinicians offer abortions at later gestation. In 2012, 95 percent of facilities offered abortions at 8 weeks' gestation, 72 percent at 12 weeks', 34 percent at 20 weeks', and 16 percent at 24 weeks' (Jerman and Jones, 2014).

According to Guttmacher's analysis, there is a sharp decline in abortion provision by nonspecialized clinics and physician's offices after 9 weeks' gestation, suggesting that these facilities are more likely to offer only early abortion services (Jerman and Jones, 2014).

Regulations That Affect Availability

In many states, abortion-specific regulations address provider education and training and the type of clinician that is permitted to provide abortion services. Many states have regulations limiting the scope of practice for APCs and excluding nonphysician providers from performing abortions (ACOG, 2014a,b; Guttmacher Institute, 2017a; O'Connell et al., 2009). In 15 states plus the District of Columbia (DC), APCs may provide medication abortions, and in 6 of those states plus DC, APCs are also permitted to perform aspiration abortions independently (Guttmacher Institute, 2017a; RHN, 2017). However, 35 states require all abortions (including medication and aspiration abortions) to be performed by a licensed physician (see Figure 3-2).

Twenty states require the involvement of a second physician if an abortion is performed after a specified gestation, typically after 22 weeks since the last menstrual period or later in the pregnancy (Guttmacher Institute, 2017b). No clinical guidelines suggest that D&E and induction abortions require the involvement of a second physician (ACOG, 2015; NAF, 2017; RCOG, 2011, 2015; SFP, 2011, 2013; WHO, 2014). One state requires the provider be either a board-certified OB/GYN or eligible for certification (Guttmacher Institute, 2017c). In one state, only an OB/GYN is permitted

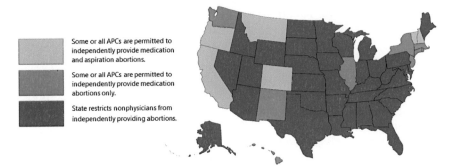

FIGURE 3-2 Regulations defining the level of provider credentialing required to provide abortions, by state and abortion method.
NOTE: APC = advanced practice clinician.
SOURCE: Adapted from RHN, 2017. Created by Samantha Andrews. Used with permission.

to provide abortions after 14 weeks' gestation (Guttmacher Institute, 2017c). By establishing higher-level credentials than are necessary based on the clinical competencies identified earlier in this chapter, these policies can reduce the availability of providers, resulting in inequitable access to abortion care based on a woman's geography. In addition, these policies can limit patients' preferences, as patient choice is contingent on the availability of trained and experienced providers (ACOG, 2015). Limiting choices impacts patient-centered care, and also negatively affects the efficiency of abortion services by potentially increasing the costs of abortion care as the result of requiring the involvement of a physician to perform a procedure that can be provided safely and effectively by an APC.

Abortion-specific regulations limit training opportunities in many states. Twelve states have laws that specifically prohibit the provision of abortion services in public institutions, such as state-run hospitals or health systems.[12] This type of restriction precludes training in those sites and can make it challenging for educational programs located in those facilities to comply with the abortion-related training requirements stipulated by academic credentialing organizations discussed earlier.

SUMMARY

This chapter has addressed several questions regarding the competencies and training of the clinical workforce that performs abortions in the United States. The committee found that abortion care, in general, requires providers skilled in patient preparation (education, counseling, and informed consent); clinical assessment (confirming intrauterine pregnancy, determining gestation, taking a relevant medical history, and physical examination); pain management; identification and management of side effects and serious complications; and contraceptive counseling and provision. To provide medication abortions, the clinician should be skilled in all these areas. To provide aspiration abortions, the clinician should also be skilled in the technical aspects of an aspiration procedure. To provide D&E abortions, the clinician needs the relevant surgical expertise and sufficient caseload to maintain the requisite surgical skills. To provide induction abortions, the clinician requires the skills needed for managing labor and delivery.

Both physicians (typically OB/GYNs and family medicine physicians, but other physicians can be trained) and APCs can provide medication

---

[12]Personal communication, O. Cappello, Guttmacher Institute, August 4, 2017: AZ § 15-1630, GA § 20-2-773; KS § 65-6733 and § 76-3308; KY § 311.800; LA RS § 40:1299 and RS § 4 0.1061; MO § 188.210 and § 188.215; MS § 41-41-91; ND § 14-02.3-04; OH § 5101.57; OK 63 § 1-741.1; PA 18 § 3215; TX § 285.202.

and aspiration abortions safely and effectively. Many states, however, prohibit nonphysicians from performing abortions regardless of the method. OB/GYNs, family medicine physicians, and other physicians with appropriate training and experience can provide D&E abortions. The committee did not find research assessing the ability of APCs, given the appropriate training, to perform D&Es safely and effectively. Induction abortions can be provided by clinicians (OB/GYNs, family medicine physicians, and CNMs) with training in managing labor and delivery.

Access to clinical education and training in abortion care in the United States is highly variable at both the undergraduate and graduate levels. Medical residents and other advanced clinical trainees often have to find abortion training and experience in settings outside of their educational program. Training opportunities are particularly limited in the Southern and Midwestern states, as well as in rural areas throughout the country.

REFERENCES

AAFP (American Academy of Family Physicians). 2016. *Recommended curriculum guidelines for family medicine residents: Women's health and gynecologic care.* AAFP reprint no. 282. http://www.aafp.org/dam/AAFP/documents/medical_education_residency/program_directors/Reprint282_Women.pdf (accessed October 19, 2017).

AAPA (American Academy of Physician Assistants). 2017. *PA: Scope of practice.* AAPA issue brief. https://www.aapa.org/wp-content/uploads/2017/01/Issue-brief_Scope-of-Practice_0117-1.pdf (accessed October 11, 2017).

ACGME (Accreditation Council for Graduate Medical Education). 2016. *Number of accredited programs academic year 2015–2016, United States.* https://apps.acgme.org/ads/Public/Reports/ReportRun?ReportId=3&CurrentYear=2016&AcademicYearId=2015 (accessed February 12, 2018).

ACGME. 2017a. *ACGME program requirements for graduate medical education in family medicine.* https://www.acgme.org/Portals/0/PFAssets/ProgramRequirements/120_family_medicine_2017-07-01.pdf?ver=2017-06-30-083354-350 (accessed December 7, 2017).

ACGME. 2017b. *ACGME program requirements for graduate medical education in obstetrics and gynecology.* http://www.acgme.org/Portals/0/PFAssets/ProgramRequirements/220_obstetrics_and_gynecology_2017-07-01.pdf (accessed October 19, 2017).

ACGME. 2017c. *Number of accredited programs academic year 2016–2017, United States.* https://apps.acgme.org/ads/Public/Reports/ReportRun?ReportId=3&CurrentYear=2017&AcademicYearId=2016 (accessed January 5, 2018).

ACNM (American College of Nurse-Midwives). 2011a. *Definition of midwifery and scope of practice of certified nurse-midwives and certified midwives.* http://www.midwife.org/ACNM/files/ACNMLibraryData/UPLOADFILENAME/000000000266/Definition%20of%20Midwifery%20and%20Scope%20of%20Practice%20of%20CNMs%20and%20CMs%20Feb%202012.pdf (accessed October 11, 2017).

ACNM. 2011b. *Position statement: Reproductive health choices.* http://midwife.org/ACNM/files/ACNMLibraryData/UPLOADFILENAME/000000000087/Reproductive_Choices.pdf (accessed February 11, 2018).

ACNM. 2011c. *Standards for the practice of midwifery.* http://www.midwife.org/ACNM/files/ACNMLibraryData/UPLOADFILENAME/000000000051/Standards_for_Practice_of_Midwifery_Sept_2011.pdf (accessed October 11, 2017).

ACNM. 2012. *Core competencies for basic midwifery practice.* http://www.midwife.org/ACNM/files/ACNMLibraryData/UPLOADFILENAME/000000000050/Core%20Comptencies%20Dec%202012.pdf (accessed October 11, 2017).

ACOG (American College of Obstetricians and Gynecologists). 2014a. *Committee opinion no. 612: Abortion training and education.* Committee on Health Care for Underserved Women. http://www.acog.org/Resources-And-Publications/Committee-Opinions/Committee-on-Health-Care-for-Underserved-Women/Abortion-Training-and-Education (accessed October 16, 2017).

ACOG. 2014b. *Committee opinion no. 613: Increasing access to abortion.* Committee on Health Care for Underserved Women. https://www.acog.org/-/media/Committee-Opinions/Committee-on-Health-Care-for-Underserved-Women/co613.pdf?dmc=1&ts=20171011T2045552523 (accessed October 16, 2017).

ACOG. 2015. Practice bulletin no. 135: Second-trimester abortion. *Obstetrics & Gynecology* 121(6):1394–1406.

ACOG and SFP (Society for Family Planning). 2014. Practice bulletin no. 143: Medical management of first-trimester abortion. *Obstetrics & Gynecology* 123(3):676–692.

Allen, R. H., and A. B. Goldberg. 2016. Cervical dilation before first-trimester surgical abortion (<14 weeks' gestation). *Contraception* 93(4):277–291.

Almeling, R., L. Tews, and S. Dudley. 2000. Abortion training in U.S. obstetrics and gynecology residency programs, 1998. *Family Planning Perspectives* 32(6):268–271, 320.

ANSIRH (Advancing New Standards in Reproductive Health). 2014. HWPP #171 final data update. *ANSIRH, Health Workforce Pilot Project,* June. https://www.ansirh.org/sites/default/files/documents/hwppupdate-june2014.pdf (accessed February 13, 2018).

APAOG (Association of Physician Assistants in Obstetrics and Gynecology). 2017. *OBGYN residency.* http://www.paobgyn.org/residency (accessed October 20, 2017).

APHA (American Public Health Association). 2011. *Provision of abortion care by advanced practice nurses and physician assistants.* https://www.apha.org/policies-and-advocacy/public-health-policy-statements/policy-database/2014/07/28/16/00/provision-of-abortion-care-by-advanced-practice-nurses-and-physician-assistants (accessed October 20, 2017).

APRN (Advanced Practice Registered Nurses) and NCSBN (National Council of State Boards of Nursing). 2008. *Consensus model for APRN regulation: Licensure, accreditation, certification and education.* Chicago, IL: National Council of State Boards of Nursing. https://www.ncsbn.org/Consensus_Model_for_APRN_Regulation_July_2008.pdf (accessed October 11, 2017).

ARC-PA (Accreditation Review Commission on Education for the Physician Assistant). 2010. *Accreditation standards for physician assistant education,* 4th ed. Johns Creek, GA: ARC-PA. http://paeaonline.org/wp-content/uploads/2016/07/12b-ARC-PA-Standards.pdf (accessed October 20, 2017).

Baird, T. L., L. D. Castleman, A. G. Hyman, R. E. Gringle, and P. D. Blumenthal. 2007. *Clinician's guide for second-trimester abortion,* 2nd ed. Chapel Hill, NC: Ipas.

Baker, A., and T. Beresford. 2009. Informed consent, patient education, and counseling. In *Management of unintended and abnormal pregnancy,* 1st ed., edited by M. Paul, E. S. Lichtenberg, L. Borgatta, D. A. Grimes, P. G. Stubblefield, and M. D. Creinin. Hoboken, NJ: Blackwell Publishing. Pp. 48–62.

Barnard, S., C. Kim, M. H. Park, and T. D. Ngo. 2015. Doctors or mid-level providers for abortion. *Cochrane Database Systematic Reviews* 27(7):CD011242.

Baum, S. E., K. White, K. Hopkins, J. E. Potter, and D. Grossman. 2016. Women's experience obtaining abortion care in Texas after implementation of restrictive abortion laws: A qualitative study. *PLoS One* 11(10):e0165048.

Beckman, L. J., S. M. Harvey, and S. J. Satre. 2002. The delivery of medical abortion services: The views of experienced providers. *Women's Health Issues* 12(2):103–112.

Bennett, I. M., M. Baylson, K. Kalkstein, G. Gillespie, S. L. Bellamy, and J. Fleischman. 2009. Early abortion in family medicine: Clinical outcomes. *Annals of Family Medicine* 7(6):527–533.

Bessett, D., K. Gorski, D. Jinadasa, M. Ostrow, and M. J. Peterson. 2011. Out of time and out of pocket: Experiences of women seeking state-subsidized insurance for abortion care in Massachusetts. *Women's Health Issues* 21(3 Suppl.):S21–S25.

Brahmi, D., C. Dehlendorf, D. Engel, K. Grumbach, C. Joffe, and M. Gold. 2007. A descriptive analysis of abortion training in family medicine residency programs. *Family Medicine* 39(6):399–403.

Creinin, M. D., and K. G. Danielsson. 2009. Medical abortion in early pregnancy. In *Management of unintended and abnormal pregnancy*, 1st ed., edited by M. Paul, E. S. Lichtenberg, L. Borgatta, D. A. Grimes, P. G. Stubblefield, and M. D. Creinin. Hoboken, NJ: Blackwell Publishing. Pp. 111–134.

Davis, A., and T. Easterling. 2009. Medical evaluation and management. In *Management of unintended and abnormal pregnancy*, 1st ed., edited by M. Paul, E. S. Lichtenberg, L. Borgatta, D. A. Grimes, P. G. Stubblefield, and M. D. Creinin. Hoboken, NJ: Blackwell Publishing. Pp. 78–79.

Dehlendorf, C., D. Brahmi, D. Engel, K. Grumbach, C. Joffe, and M. Gold. 2007. Integrating abortion training into family medicine residency programs. *Family Medicine* 39(5):337–342.

Drey, E. A., D. G. Foster, R. A. Jackson, S. J. Lee, L. H. Cardenas, and P. D. Darney. 2006. Risk factors associated with presenting for abortion in the second trimester. *Obstetrics & Gynecology* 107(1):128–135.

Eastwood, K. L., J. E. Kacmar, J. Steinauer, S. Weitzen, and L. A. Boardman. 2006. Abortion training in United States obstetrics and gynecology residency programs. *Obstetrics & Gynecology* 108(2):303–308.

FDA (U.S. Food and Drug Administration). 2016. *Highlights of prescribing information: Mifeprex®* (revised 3/2016). https://www.accessdata.fda.gov/drugsatfda_docs/label/2016/020687s020lbl.pdf (accessed October 20, 2017).

FFP (Fellowship in Family Planning). 2017. *Where are the fellowships located?* https://www.familyplanningfellowship.org/fellowship-programs (accessed October 20, 2017).

Finer, L. B., L. F. Frohwirth, L. A. Dauphinee, S. Singh, and A. M. Moore. 2006. Timing of steps and reasons for delays in obtaining abortions in the United States. *Contraception* 74(4):334–344.

Foster, A. M., P. Chelsea, M. K. Allee, K. Simmonds, M. Zurek, and A. Brown. 2006. Abortion education in nurse practitioner, physician assistant and certified nurse-midwifery programs: A national survey. *Contraception* 73(4):408–414.

Foster, D. G., and K. Kimport. 2013. Who seeks abortions at or after 20 weeks? *Perspectives on Sexual and Reproductive Health* 45(4):210–218.

Freedman, L. R., and D. B. Stulberg. 2013. Conflicts in care for obstetric complications in Catholic hospitals. *AJOB Primary Research* 4(4):1–10.

Freedman, L. R., U. Landy, and J. Steinauer. 2008. When there's a heartbeat: Miscarriage management in Catholic-owned hospitals. *American Journal of Public Health* 98(10):1774–1778.

French, V., R. Anthony, C. Souder, C. Geistkemper, E. Drey, and J. Steinauer. 2016. Influence of clinician referral on Nebraska women's decision-to-abortion time. *Contraception* 93(3):236–243.

Fuentes, L., S. Lebenkoff, K. White, C. Gerdts, K. Hopkins, J. E. Potter, and D. Grossman. 2016. Women's experiences seeking abortion care shortly after the closure of clinics due to a restrictive law in Texas. *Contraception* 93(4):292–297.

Gavin, L., S. Moskosky, M. Carter, K. Curtis, E. Glass, E. Godfrey, A. Marcell, N. Mautone-Smith, K. Pazol, N. Tepper, and L. Zapata. 2014. Providing quality family planning services: Recommendations of CDC and the U.S. Office of Population Affairs. *Morbidity and Mortality Weekly Reports* 63(RR04):1–29. Atlanta, GA: Centers for Disease Control and Prevention. https://www.cdc.gov/mmwr/preview/mmwrhtml/rr6304a1.htm (accessed September 15, 2017).

Gemzell-Danielsson, K., and S. Lalitkumar. 2008. Second trimester medical abortion with mifepristone-misoprostol and misoprostol alone: A review of methods and management. *Reproductive Health Matters* 16(31 Suppl.):162–172.

Gerdts, C., L. Fuentes, D. Grossman, K. White, B. Keefe-Oates, S. E. Baum, K. Hopkins, C. W. Stolp, and J. E. Potter. 2016. Impact of clinic closures on women obtaining abortion services after implementation of a restrictive law in Texas. *American Journal of Public Health* 106(5):857–864.

Goldman, M. B., J. S. Occhiuto, L. E. Peterson, J. G. Zapka, and R. H. Palmer. 2004. Physician assistants as providers of surgically induced abortion services. *American Journal of Public Health* 94(8):1352–1357.

Goldstein, S. R., and M. F. Reeves. 2009. Clinical assessment and ultrasound in early pregnancy. In *Management of unintended and abnormal pregnancy*, 1st ed., edited by M. Paul, E. S. Lichtenberg, L. Borgatta, D. A. Grimes, P. G. Stubblefield, and M. D. Creinin. Hoboken, NJ: Blackwell Publishing. Pp. 63–77.

Goodman, S., G. Shih, M. Hawkins, S. Feierabend, P. Lossy, N. J. Waxman, M. Gold, and C. Dehlendorf. 2013. A long-term evaluation of a required reproductive health training rotation with opt-out provisions for family medicine residents. *Family Medicine* 45(3):180–186.

Goodman, S., G. Flaxman, and TEACH Trainers Collaborative Working Group. 2016. *Teach early abortion training workbook*, 5th ed. San Francisco, CA: UCSF Bixby Center for Global Reproductive Health. http://www.teachtraining.org/training-tools/early-abortion-training-workbook (accessed October 20, 2017).

Grossman, D., K. Blanchard, and P. Blumenthal. 2008. Complications after second trimester surgical and medical abortion. *Reproductive Health Matters* 16(31 Suppl.):173–182.

Grossman, D., S. Baum, L. Fuentes, K. White, K. Hopkins, A. Stevenson, and J. E. Potter. 2014. Change in abortion services after implementation of a restrictive law in Texas. *Contraception* 90(5):496–501.

Grossman, D., K. White, K. Hopkins, and J. E. Potter. 2017. Change in distance to nearest facility and abortion in Texas, 2012 to 2014. *Journal of the American Medical Association* 317(4):437–438.

Guttmacher Institute. 2017a. *An overview of abortion laws*. Washington, DC: Guttmacher Institute. https://www.guttmacher.org/state-policy/explore/overview-abortion-laws (accessed October 20, 2017).

Guttmacher Institute. 2017b. *State policies on later abortions*. Washington, DC: Guttmacher Institute. https://www.guttmacher.org/state-policy/explore/state-policies-later-abortions (accessed September 21, 2017).

Guttmacher Institute. 2017c. *Targeted regulation of abortion providers*. Washington, DC: Guttmacher Institute. https://www.guttmacher.org/state-policy/explore/targeted-regulation-abortion-providers (accessed June 23, 2017).

Hammond, C., and S. Chasen. 2009. Dilation and evacuation. In *Management of unintended and abnormal pregnancy*, 1st ed., edited by M. Paul, E. S. Lichtenberg, L. Borgatta, D. A. Grimes, P. G. Stubblefield, and M. D. Creinin. Hoboken, NJ: Blackwell Publishing. Pp. 157–177.

Health IT. 2013. *Shared decision making*. https://www.healthit.gov/sites/default/files/nlc_shared_decision_making_fact_sheet.pdf (accessed January 10, 2018).

Herbitter, C., M. Greenberg, J. Fletcher, C. Query, J. Dalby, and M. Gold. 2011. Family planning training in U.S. family medicine residencies. *Family Medicine* 43(8):574–581.

Herbitter, C., A. Bennett, D. Finn, D. Schubert, I. M. Bennett, and M. Gold. 2013. Management of early pregnancy failure and induced abortion by family medicine educators. *Journal of the American Board of Family Medicine* 26(6):751–758.

Hern, W. M. 2016. *Second-trimester surgical abortion.* https://www.glowm.com/section_view/heading/Second-Trimester%20Surgical%20Abortion/item/441 (accessed October 6, 2017).

ICM (International Confederation of Midwives). 2011a. *Global standards for midwifery regulation.* The Hague, Netherlands: ICM. http://internationalmidwives.org/assets/uploads/documents/Global%20Standards%20Competencies%20Tools/English/GLOBAL%20STANDARDS%20FOR%20MIDWIFERY%20REGULATION%20ENG.pdf (accessed October 20, 2017).

ICM. 2011b. *Position statement: Midwives' provision of abortion-related services.* https://internationalmidwives.org/assets/uploads/documents/Position%20Statements%20-%20English/Reviewed%20PS%20in%202014/PS2008_011%20V2014%20Midwives'%20provision%20of%20abortion%20related%20services%20ENG.pdf (accessed February 11, 2018).

ICM. 2013. *Essential competencies for basic midwifery practice, 2010 (revised 2013).* The Hague, Netherlands: ICM. https://internationalmidwives.org/assets/uploads/documents/CoreDocuments/ICM%20Essential%20Competencies%20for%20Basic%20Midwifery%20Practice%202010,%20revised%202013.pdf (accessed February 12, 2018).

Jackson, C. B., and A. M. Foster. 2012. OB/GYN training in abortion care: Results from a national survey. *Contraception* 86(4):407–412.

Janiak, E., I. Kawachi, A. Goldberg, and B. Gottlieb. 2014. Abortion barriers and perceptions of gestational age among women seeking abortion care in the latter half of the second trimester. *Contraception* 89(4):322–327.

Jatlaoui, T. C., A. Ewing, M. G. Mandel, K. B. Simmons, D. B. Suchdev, D. J. Jamieson, and K. Pazol. 2016. Abortion surveillance—United States, 2013. *MMWR Surveillance Summaries* 65(SS-12):1–44.

Jerman, J., and R. K. Jones. 2014. Secondary measures of access to abortion services in the United States, 2011 and 2012: Gestational age limits, cost, and harassment. *Women's Health Issues* 24(4):e419–e424.

Johns, N. E., D. G. Foster, and U. D. Upadhyay. 2017. Distance traveled for Medicaid-covered abortion care in California. *BMC Health Services Research* 17(287):1–11.

Jones, R. K., and J. Jerman. 2013. How far did U.S. women travel for abortion services in 2008? *Journal of Women's Health* 22(8):706–713.

Jones, R. K., and J. Jerman. 2014. Abortion incidence and service availability in the United States, 2011. *Perspectives on Sexual and Reproductive Health* 46(1):3–14.

Jones, R. K., and J. Jerman. 2016. *Time to appointment and delays in accessing care among U.S. abortion patients.* Washington, DC: Guttmacher Institute. https://www.guttmacher.org/report/delays-in-accessing-care-among-us-abortion-patients (accessed April 15, 2017).

Jones, R. K., and J. Jerman. 2017a. Abortion incidence and service availability in the United States, 2014. *Perspectives on Sexual and Reproductive Health* 49(1):17–27.

Jones, R. K., and J. Jerman. 2017b. Characteristics and circumstances of U.S. women who obtain very early and second trimester abortions. *PLoS One* 12(1):e0169969.

Kapp, N., and H. von Hertzen. 2009. Medical methods to induce abortion in the second trimester. In *Management of unintended and abnormal pregnancy*, 1st ed., edited by M. Paul, E. S. Lichtenberg, L. Borgatta, D. A. Grimes, P. G. Stubblefield, and M. D. Creinin. Hoboken, NJ: Blackwell Publishing. Pp. 178–192.

Kiley, J. W., L. M. Yee, C. M. Niemi, J. M. Feinglass, and M. A. Simon. 2010. Delays in request for pregnancy termination: Comparison of patients in the first and second trimesters. *Contraception* 81(5):446–451.

Kopp Kallner, H., R. Gomperts, E. Salomonsson, M. Johansson, L. Marions, and K. Gem-zell-Danielsson. 2015. The efficacy, safety, and acceptability of medical termination of pregnancy provided by standard care by doctors or by nurse-midwives: A randomised controlled equivalence trial. *British Journal of Obstetricians and Gynaecologists* 122(4):510–517.

Lesnewski, R., L. Prine, and M. Gold. 2003. Abortion training as an integral part of residency training. *Family Medicine* 35(6):469–471.

Levi, A., J. E. Angel, and D. Taylor. 2012. Midwives and abortion care: A model for achieving competency. *Journal of Midwifery & Women's Health* 57(3):285–289.

Lohr, P. A., J. L. Hayes, and K. Gemzell-Danielsson. 2008. Surgical versus medical methods for second trimester induced abortion. *Cochrane Database of Systematic Reviews* (1):CD006714.

Lyus, R. J., P. Gianutsos, and M. Gold. 2009. First trimester procedural abortion in family medicine. *Journal of the American Board of Family Medicine* 22(2):169–174.

MAP (Midwest Access Project). 2017. *What we do.* http://midwestaccessproject.org/what-we-do (accessed October 20, 2017).

McLemore, M. R., S. Desai, L. Freedman, E. A. James, and D. Taylor. 2014. Women know best—findings from a thematic analysis of 5,214 surveys of abortion care experience. *Women's Health Issues* 24(6):594–599.

Meckstroth, K., and M. Paul. 2009. First-trimester aspiration abortion. In *Management of unintended and abnormal pregnancy*, 1st ed., edited by M. Paul, E. S. Lichtenberg, L. Borgatta, D. A. Grimes, P. G. Stubblefield, and M. D. Creinin. Hoboken, NJ: Blackwell Publishing. Pp. 135–156.

NAF (National Abortion Federation). 2017. *Clinical policy guidelines for abortion care.* Washington, DC: NAF.

NAF and CFC (Clinicians for Choice). 2018. *Role of CNMs, NPs, and PAs in abortion care.* https://5aa1b2xfmfh2e2mk03kk8rsx-wpengine.netdna-ssl.com/wp-content/uploads/CNM_NP_PA_org_statements.pdf (accessed February 11, 2018).

Nanda, K., L. M. Lopez, D. A. Grimes, A. Peloggia, and G. Nanda. 2012. Expectant care versus surgical treatment for miscarriage (review). *Cochrane Database of Systemic Reviews* 3:CD003518.

Newmann, S. J., A. Dalve-Endres, and E. A. Drey. 2008. Clinical guidelines: Cervical preparation for surgical abortion from 20 to 24 weeks' gestation. *Society of Family Planning* 77(4):308–314.

Newmann, S. J., A. Dalve-Endres, J. T. Diedrich, J. E. Steinauer, K. Meckstroth, and E. A. Drey. 2010. Cervical preparation for second trimester dilation and evacuation. *Cochrane Database of Systematic Reviews* 8:CD007310.

Ngo, T. D., M. H. Park, and C. Free. 2013. Safety and effectiveness of termination services performed by doctors versus midlevel providers: A systematic review and analysis. *International Journal of Women's Health* 5:9–17.

Nichols, M., B. Halvofrson-Boyd, R. C. Goldstein, C. M. Gevirtz, and D. Healow. 2009. Pain management. In *Management of unintended and abnormal pregnancy: Comprehensive abortion care*, 1st ed., edited by M. Paul, E. S. Lichtenberg, L. Borgatta, D. A. Grimes, P. G. Stubblefield, and M. D. Creinin. Hoboken, NJ: Wiley-Blackwell. Pp. 90–110.

NONPF (Nurse Organization of Nurse Practitioners Faculties). 2017. *Nurse practitioner core competencies content.* http://c.ymcdn.com/sites/www.nonpf.org/resource/resmgr/competencies/2017_NPCoreComps_with_Curric.pdf (accessed October 20, 2017).

Nothnagle, M., J. M. Sicilia, S. Forman, J. Fish, W. Ellert, R. Gebhard, B. F. Kelly, J. L. Pfenninger, M. Tuggy, W. M. Rodney, and STFM Group on Hospital Medicine and Procedural Training. 2008. Required procedural training in family medicine residency: A consensus statement. *Family Medicine* 40(4):248–252.

O'Connell, K., H. E. Jones, E. S. Lichtenberg, and M. Paul. 2008. Second-trimester surgical abortion practices: A survey of National Abortion Federation members. *Contraception* 78(6):492–499.

O'Connell, K., H. E. Jones, M. Simon, V. Saporta, M. N. Paul, M. E., and S. Lichtenberg. 2009. First-trimester surgical abortion practices: A survey of National Abortion Federation members. *Contraception* 79(5):385–392.

Ostrach, B., and M. Cheyney. 2014. Navigating social and institutional obstacles: Low-income women seeking abortion. *Quality Health Research* 24(7):1006–1017.

Paul, M., and M. E. Norton. 2016. Ensuring access to safe, legal abortion in an increasingly complex regulatory environment. *Obstetrics & Gynecology* 128(1):171–175.

Paul, M., K. Nobel, S. Goodman, P. Lossy, J. E. Moschella, and H. Hammer. 2007. Abortion training in three family medicine programs: Resident and patient outcomes. *Family Medicine* 39(3):184–189.

Prine, L., R. Lesnewski, N. Berley, and M. Gold. 2003. Medical abortion in family practice: A case series. *Journal of the American Board of Family Medicine* 16(4):290–295.

Prine, L., C. Shannon, G. Gillespie, W. A. Crowden, J. Fortin, M. Howe, and I. Dzuba. 2010. Medical abortion: Outcomes in a family medicine setting. *Journal of the American Board of Family Medicine* 23(4):509–513.

RCOG (Royal College of Obstetricians and Gynaecologists). 2011. *The care of women requesting induced abortion* (Evidence-based clinical guideline number 7). London, UK: RCOG Press.

RCOG. 2015. *Best practice in comprehensive abortion care* (Best practice paper no. 7). London, UK: RCOG Press.

Renner, R.-M., D. Brahmi, and N. Kapp. 2013. Who can provide effective and safe termination of pregnancy care? A systematic review. *British Journal of Obstetrics and Gynecology* 120(1):23–31.

RHEDI (Reproductive Health Education in Family Medicine). 2017. *Family medicine residencies with abortion training.* http://www.rhedi.org/education/residency-training/#rhediprograms (accessed October 20, 2017).

RHN (Reproductive Health in Nursing). 2017. *Providing abortion care: A professional toolkit for nurse-midwives, nurse practitioners, and physician assistants.* https://rhnursing.org/resource/abortion-provider-toolkit-nurses (accessed October 20, 2017).

Roberts, S. C., H. Gould, K. Kimport, T. A. Weitz, and D. G. Foster. 2014. Out-of-pocket costs and insurance coverage for abortion in the United States. *Women's Health Issues* 24(2):e211–e218.

Rubin, S. E., J. Fletcher, T. Stein, P. Segall-Gutierrez, and M. Gold. 2011. Determinants of intrauterine contraception provision among U.S. family physicians: A national survey of knowledge, attitudes, and practice. *Contraception* 83(5):472–478.

Ryan Residency Training Program. 2017a. *About the Ryan Program.* https://www.ryanprogram.org/about-ryan-program (accessed October 20, 2017).

Ryan Residency Training Program. 2017b. *Map and locations of Ryan Program sites.* https://www.ryanprogram.org/map-and-locations (accessed October 20, 2017).

Ryan Residency Training Program. 2017c. *Ryan Program didactics.* https://ryanprogram.org/sites/default/files/Ryan%20Program%20Milestones.pdf (accessed October 20, 2017).

SFP (Society of Family Planning). 2011. Labor induction abortion in the second trimester. *Contraception* 84(1):4–18.

SFP. 2013. Interruption of nonviable pregnancies of 24–28 weeks' gestation using medical methods. *Contraception* 88(3):341–349.

SFP. 2014. Cervical preparation for second-trimester surgical abortion prior to 20 weeks' gestation. *Contraception* 89(2):75–84.

Simmonds, K. E., M. W. Beal, and M. K. Eagen-Torkko. 2017. Updates to the U.S. Food and Drug Administration regulations for Mifepristone: Implications for clinical practice and access to abortion care. *Journal of Midwifery & Women's Health* 62(3):348–352.

Sjöström, S., M. Dragoman, M. S. Fønhus, B. Ganatra, and K. Gemzell-Danielsson. 2017. Effectiveness, safety, and acceptability of first-trimester medical termination of pregnancy performed by non-doctor providers: A systematic review. *British Journal of Obstetrics and Gynaecology* 124(13):1928–1940.

Steinauer, J., T. DePineres, A. Robert, J. Westfall, and P. Darney. 1997. Training family practice residents in abortion and other reproductive health care: A nationwide survey. *Family Planning Perspectives* 29(5):222–227.

Steinauer, J., C. Dehlendorf, K. Grumbach, U. Landy, and P. Darney. 2012. Multi-specialty family planning training: Collaborating to meet the needs of women. *Contraception* 86(3):188–190.

Steinauer, J. E., M. Hawkins, J. K. Turk, P. Darney, F. Preskill, and U. Landy. 2013a. Opting out of abortion training: Benefits of partial participation in a dedicated family planning rotation for OB-GYN residents. *Contraception* 87(1):88–92.

Steinauer, J. E., J. K. Turk, M. C. Fulton, K. H. Simonson, and U. Landy. 2013b. The benefits of family planning training: A 10-year review of the Ryan Residency Training Program. *Contraception* 88(2):275–280.

Stubblefield, P. G., S. Carr-Ellis, and L. Borgatta. 2004. Methods for induced abortion. *Obstetrics & Gynecology* 104(1):174–185.

Stulberg, D. B., A. M. Dude, I. Dahlquist, and F. A. Curlin. 2011. Abortion provision among practicing obstetrician-gynecologists. *Obstetrics & Gynecology* 118(3):609–614.

Stulberg, D. B., R. A. Jackson, and L. R. Freedman. 2016. Referrals for services prohibited in Catholic health care facilities. *Perspectives on Sexual and Reproductive Health* 48(3):111–117.

Summit, A. K., and M. Gold. 2017. The effects of abortion training on family medicine residents' clinical experience. *Family Medicine* 49(1):22–27.

Summit, A. K., L. M. J. Casey, A. H. Bennett, A. Karasz, and M. Gold. 2016. "I don't want to go anywhere else": Patient experiences of abortion in family medicine. *Family Medicine* 48(1):30–34.

Talley, P., and G. Bergus. 1996. Abortion training in family practice residency programs. *Family Medicine* 28(4):245–248.

Taylor, D., B. Safriet, G. Dempsey, B. Kruse, and C. Jackson. 2009. *Providing abortion care: A professional toolkit for nurse-midwives, nurse practitioners, and physician assistants.* San Francisco, CA: ANSIRH. http://apctoolkit.org/wp-content/themes/apctoolkit/index.html (accessed October 20, 2017).

Taylor, D., D. Postlethwaite, S. Desai, E. A. James, A. W. Calhoun, K. Sheehan, and T. A. Weitz. 2013. Multiple determinants of the abortion care experience: From the patient's perspective. *American Journal of Medical Quality* 28(6):510–518.

Tocce, K., and B. Severson. 2012. Funding for abortion training in OB/GYN residency. *American Medical Association Journal of Ethics* 14(2):112–117.

Turk, J. K., F. Preskill, U. Landy, C. H. Rocca, and J. E. Steinauer. 2014. Availability and characteristics of abortion training in U.S. OB-GYN residency programs: A national survey. *Contraception* 89(4):271–277.

Upadhyay, U. D., T. A. Weitz, R. K. Jones, R. E. Barar, and D. G. Foster. 2014. Denial of abortion because of provider gestational age limits in the United States. *American Journal of Public Health* 104(9):1687–1694.

Upadhyay, U. D., N. E. Johns, K. R. Meckstroth, and J. L. Kerns. 2017. Distance traveled for an abortion and source of care after abortion. *Obstetrics & Gynecology* 130(3):616–624.

Weitz, T. A., D. Taylor, S. Desai, U. D. Upadhyay, J. Waldman, M. F. Battistelli, and E. A. Drey. 2013. Safety of aspiration abortion performed by nurse practitioners, certified nurse midwives, and physician assistants under a California legal waiver. *American Journal of Public Health* 103(3):454–461.

White, K., V. deMartelly, D. Grossman, and J. M. Turan. 2016. Experiences accessing abortion care in Alabama among women traveling for services. *Women's Health Issues* 26(3):298–304.

WHO (World Health Organization). 2012. *Safe abortion: Technical and policy guidance for health systems*. Geneva, Switzerland: WHO.

WHO. 2014. *Clinical practice handbook for safe abortion*. Geneva, Switzerland: WHO.

WHO. 2015. *Health worker roles in providing safe abortion care and post-abortion contraception*. Geneva, Switzerland: WHO.

Woodcock, J. 2016. Letter from the director of the FDA Center for Drug Evaluation and Research to Donna Harrison, Gene Rudd, and Penny Young Nance. Re: Docket No. FDA-2002-P-0364. Silver Spring, MD: U.S. Food and Drug Administration.

Wu, J. P., E. M. Godfrey, L. Prine, K. L. Anderson, H. MacNaughton, and M. Gold. 2015. Women's satisfaction with abortion care in academic family medicine centers. *Family Medicine* 47(2):98–106.

4

Long-Term Health Effects

When evaluating the safety of any medical intervention, it is important not only to consider the immediate potential complications but also to evaluate the potential for associated long-term health effects. Research on abortion's potential long-term health consequences has focused on reproductive and mental health outcomes, as well as other outcomes including breast cancer risk and premature death. This chapter reviews research on the long-term physical and mental health effects of having an abortion.[1] The focus is on four putative areas of potential harm:

- future childbearing and pregnancy outcomes (e.g., secondary infertility; ectopic pregnancy; spontaneous abortion and stillbirth; complications of pregnancy; and preterm birth, small for gestational age, and low birthweight);
- risk of breast cancer;
- mental health disorders; and
- premature death.

---

[1]This chapter reviews the epidemiological research on abortion's long-term physical and mental health effects. In epidemiology, an odds ratio is the statistic used by researchers to measure the association between an "exposure" (e.g., a prior abortion) and an outcome of interest. Odds ratios compare the relative odds of a particular health outcome, given the exposure, and can indicate whether the exposure is a risk factor, as well as the magnitude of the risk. The confidence interval (CI) indicates the precision of the estimate.

As noted in Chapter 1, some states require that abortion patients be offered or provided information indicating that abortion negatively affects future fertility (Arizona, Kansas, Nebraska, North Carolina, South Dakota, and Texas); risk of breast cancer (Arkansas, Kansas, Mississippi, Oklahoma, and Texas); and/or mental health disorders (Idaho, Kansas, Louisiana, Michigan, Nebraska, North Carolina, North Dakota, Oklahoma, South Dakota, Texas, Utah, and West Virginia).[2] Some observers have also questioned whether abortion may lead to premature death (Reardon et al., 2002).

This chapter first describes the limitations of the abortion literature and the committee's criteria for identifying scientifically valid research on abortion's long-term health consequences. The remainder of the chapter presents the committee's review of what is known about each of the above putative harms of abortion.

LIMITATIONS OF THE LITERATURE

While randomized controlled trials are the gold standard research design for assessing the health effects of a medical intervention, they are not appropriate for studies assessing the long-term risks of abortion. Women seeking an abortion cannot be randomized to an experimental group that has the abortion or a control group that does not have the abortion. Researchers must use observational study designs (e.g., cohort, case control, and cross-sectional studies) to examine abortion's long-term potential for harm. However, the risk of bias is greater for observational studies than for randomized studies, and it is imperative that published studies be assessed for potential sources of bias that might affect their findings (IOM, 2011). In research, bias refers to systematic error in a study's design or execution that leads to an incorrect result (Cochrane Collaboration, 2018).

Sources of Bias

Observational studies of abortion's long-term health effects have two important sources of information bias: selective recall bias and selection bias. Each is described below.

Selective Recall Bias

Several studies have demonstrated underreporting of past abortions in surveys of American women (Beral et al., 2004; Jones and Kost, 2007; Steinberg et al., 2011). Women who have had an abortion have a tendency

---

[2]See Chapter 1, Table 1-1.

not to recall—or not to report—having had an abortion when asked (Anderson et al., 1994; Bouyer et al., 2003; Hogue, 1975; Jones and Kost, 2007; Lindefors-Harris et al., 1991). Jones and Kost (2007) pooled data from the 1997 to 2001 annual National Survey of Family Growth to assess the accuracy of women's reports of the number of their past pregnancies and the timing and outcome of each pregnancy. Data were collected from face-to-face interviews and computer-assisted, self-administered question-naires. Tallies of the survey responses were compared with national esti-mates of the number of abortions performed during the time period. Over-all, the number of self-reported abortions was only 47 percent of the total estimated number of abortions performed in the United States during the study period. Inconsistencies also were seen between women's responses during the interviews and on the self-administered questionnaire.

The committee found that selective recall bias—which occurs when there are systematic differences in study subjects' reporting of a past expo-sure (e.g., a prior abortion)—affects much of the published research on abortion's long-term health effects.[3] In case control studies, for example, subjects who had a particular negative health outcome may be more likely to report having had the past exposure compared with subjects who also had the exposure but did not have the outcome. As a consequence, healthy subjects with an exposure are more likely than unhealthy subjects to be mistakenly assigned to a nonexposure study group. When this occurs, a study is likely to conclude erroneously that the negative health outcome is associated with the exposure. Many published abortion studies are flawed in this way because women who have had an abortion are less likely to report their prior abortion if they have not experienced a long-term adverse health outcome. Such selective recall bias was first documented in a 1975 study of low-birthweight births among women who had had an abortion (Hogue, 1975) and has been demonstrated in other studies of abortion's long-term effects (Anderson et al., 1994; Bouyer et al., 2003; Lindefors-Harris et al., 1991).

Recall bias is best addressed by using registry or medical record data to document prior abortions and link the abortion histories with reliable records of subsequent patient outcomes.

---

[3]Selective (or differential) recall bias has a different effect on study results relative to general (or nondifferential) recall bias. Nondifferential recall bias occurs when all study subjects are equally likely to misrecall an exposure. When this happens, study results are likely to under-report the association between the exposure and the health outcome (Alexander et al., 2015). In studies of abortion recall and health outcomes, only differential bias has been documented. This suggests that studies that rely on women's reports of abortion and that find no associa-tion with the condition under study might be used to conclude that there is evidence of no true association. However, the committee did not utilize this assumption, but rather relied exclusively on studies that document the subjects' abortion history.

Selection Bias (Comparability of Study Populations)

Selection bias occurs when one of the baseline characteristics of the study population is associated with the outcome of interest (e.g., future pregnancy and birth complications after abortion). In such circumstances, the statistical analysis should take into account (or "control for") the differences in the prevalence of the confounding factors in the study and control groups. If the objective of a study is to determine whether having an abortion raises the risk of future mental health problems, for example, the study should control for women's mental health status at baseline (i.e., before they have the abortion). This is particularly important in mental health research because women who have an abortion report higher rates of mental health disorders *before* undergoing the procedure compared with women who give birth (Steinberg et al., 2014). Other confounding variables that may affect future health and pregnancy outcomes include socioeconomic status, race and ethnicity, smoking, and substance use. Much of the research on abortion's long-term effects has been conducted outside the United States, and a substantial volume of literature is based on abortion care in countries where such factors as socioeconomic conditions, culture, population health, health care resources, and/or the health care system are markedly different from those in the United States. In addition to the other selection criteria listed below, the committee determined the applicability of published research based on the likelihood that the abortion interventions examined reflected contemporary abortion care in the United States (e.g., in European countries). Although the committee identified studies of long-term health effects in Africa, China, India, Taiwan, and Vietnam, these studies were excluded.

The Committee's Selection Criteria

The committee's literature search strategy for this chapter is provided in Appendix D. The bibliographies of retrieved articles were reviewed to find additional relevant research. Each identified article was reviewed to determine whether the study met the criteria listed below. The findings reported in this chapter draw solely on studies that met these criteria:

- for the study population, there was objective medical record or patient registry documentation of a prior induced abortion (excluding spontaneous abortion or miscarriage);
- the study population (women with a documented abortion) was compared with a control group of women with no documented abortion history;
- the analysis controlled for mental health status prior to the abortion (if assessing the mental health effects of abortion);

- the study was published in 2000 or later and included abortions performed in 1980 or later (to help ensure that reported outcomes reflected contemporary abortion methods); and
- the clinical settings and care delivery were similar to those in the United States.

FUTURE CHILDBEARING AND PREGNANCY OUTCOMES

Many women are likely to desire and experience a future pregnancy after having had an abortion. Abortion has been investigated for its potential effect on secondary infertility; ectopic pregnancy; spontaneous abortion and stillbirth; pregnancy complications that can lead to adverse maternal or fetal health; and preterm birth, low birthweight, and/or weight that is small for gestational age. This section reviews this research.

Secondary Infertility

Does Abortion Increase the Risk of Secondary Infertility?

Secondary infertility is defined as difficulty conceiving a pregnancy or carrying a pregnancy to term after a previous pregnancy. The committee found one study on abortion and risk of secondary infertility that met its selection criteria. Holmlund and colleagues (2016) examined the pregnancy-related outcomes of 57,406 first-time mothers in Finland who gave birth between 2008 and 2010; 5,167 of the women had had a prior abortion. Using national registry data, the researchers linked the mothers' birth records with records documenting a prior abortion and/or subsequent treatment for infertility. First-time mothers with a prior abortion were significantly *less* likely to be treated for infertility compared with women in their first pregnancy (1.95 versus 5.14 percent, p <.0001), thus suggesting that there is no association between abortion and secondary infertility.

Ectopic Pregnancy

Does Abortion Increase the Risk of Ectopic Pregnancy?

An ectopic pregnancy occurs when a fertilized egg grows outside of the uterus, most commonly in a fallopian tube. As the pregnancy progresses, the fallopian tube may rupture, causing major internal bleeding (ACOG, 2017). In 2013, an estimated 0.68 percent of commercially insured pregnant women and 0.57 percent of Medicaid-insured women in the United States were diagnosed and treated for an ectopic pregnancy (Tao et al., 2017). Women with a history of upper genital tract infection (e.g., in the uterus or fallopian tubes) are at increased risk of an ectopic pregnancy (Sivalingam et al., 2011). As noted in Chapter 2, serious infection after an abortion is rare and has become even rarer since antibiotic prophylaxis became standard practice. If untreated, an abortion-related infection may increase the risk of subsequent ectopic pregnancy.

While several literature reviews have concluded that abortion is not associated with increased risk of ectopic pregnancy (Lowit et al., 2010; RCOG, 2011b; Thorp et al., 2003), all the published reviews are methodologically flawed because they include studies based on maternal recall and/ or rely heavily on studies of abortions performed before the introduction of contemporary abortion methods. The committee could identify no primary literature without these limitations.

Spontaneous Abortion (Miscarriage) and Stillbirth

Does Abortion Increase the Risk of Spontaneous Abortion and Stillbirth?

Spontaneous abortion, also referred to as miscarriage, is the spontaneous death of a fetus prior to 20 weeks' gestation. Stillbirth refers to spontaneous fetal death after 20 weeks' gestation (ODPHP, 2017). Several literature reviews have concluded that abortion is not associated with increased risk of either spontaneous abortion or stillbirth (Lowit et al., 2010; RCOG, 2011b; Thorp et al., 2003). However, as in the published reviews of abortion and subsequent ectopic pregnancy, these literature reviews include studies of abortions performed with outdated methods and are methodologically flawed by reliance on studies based on maternal recall (rather than objective documentation of an abortion). The committee could identify no relevant primary literature without these limitations, and thus was unable to draw a conclusion regarding the association between abortion and risk of spontaneous abortion and stillbirth.

Pregnancy Complications

The committee identified three primary research studies[4] that used documented records of receipt of an abortion to assess the effect of abortion

---

[4]The committee identified a fourth study that used Danish registry data to assess the effects of abortions performed from 1980 to 1982 on subsequent pregnancy complications. This study, by Zhou and colleagues (2001), was excluded from the committee's review because it is unlikely to reflect the outcomes of contemporary abortion methods. The authors report that almost all (99.7 percent) of the abortion procedures included in the study were followed by curettage. As noted in Chapter 2, sharp-metal curettage is no longer recommended because it is associated with risk of injury (NAF, 2017; RCOG, 2011b, 2015; Roblin, 2014; SFP, 2013; WHO, 2012).

on the risk of complications in a future pregnancy. The study findings are summarized below. Study details, including adjusted odds ratios (aORs), sample sizes, and the years in which the abortions occurred, are provided in Table 4-1.

In a retrospective cohort study, Jackson and colleagues (2007) linked medical records and obstetrics databases in two Chicago-area hospitals to compare the pregnancy outcomes of women who had and had not previously received a dilation and evacuation (D&E) abortion. Holmlund and colleagues (2016) linked Finnish birth and abortion registry data to compare the first full-term pregnancies of women with and without a prior abortion. Finally, Woolner and colleagues (2014) used Scottish registry data to compare the risk of preterm delivery and other birth outcomes among women with and without a prior abortion. This latter analysis has a number of strengths not characteristic of most of the available research on abortion and subsequent birth outcomes. The researchers had a large enough sample and sufficient data to control for maternal age, socioeconomic variables, weeks' gestation (≤13 weeks versus >13 weeks), and smoking, as well as to stratify the sample by type of abortion (e.g., medication versus aspiration). The study population groups included 3,186 women with a documented termination of their first pregnancy and 42,446 primigravid women.[5]

Does Abortion Increase the Risk of Hypertension of Pregnancy?

Hypertension of pregnancy includes preeclampsia and chronic and gestational hypertension. It is associated with increased risk of both maternal complications, such as placental abruption and gestational diabetes, and poor birth outcomes, such as preterm birth, having a baby that is small for gestational age, and infant death (CDC, 2016). Hypertension complicates about 5 to 10 percent of pregnancies (Garovic and August, 2013). The Woolner et al. (2014) and Holmlund et al. (2014) studies described above compared the subsequent pregnancies of women who had had prior abortions and women in their first pregnancy (without prior abortions) and found no increased risk of hypertension in pregnancy or preeclampsia among the women with prior abortions. In the Woolner et al. (2014) study, women who had had an abortion had a *lower* risk of hypertensive disease relative to women in their first pregnancy. This finding persisted when the outcomes were analyzed by type of abortion (i.e., medication and aspiration). The authors also found that the timing of abortion had no impact on hypertensive disease. Women who had undergone both early and late abortions had a *lower* risk of hypertension in pregnancy compared with women

---

[5]"Primigravid" refers to women who are pregnant for the first time.

TABLE 4-1 Studies Assessing the Association Between Abortion and Subsequent Pregnancy Complications Using Record-Linkage Methods

Author (year)	Location (time period)	Abortion Group	Comparison Group
Holmlund et al. (2016)	Finland (1983–2007)	All methods n = 5,167	Primigravid n = 52,239
Woolner et al. (2014)	Scotland (1986–2010)	All methods n = 3,186	Primigravid n = 42,446
		Aspiration n = 1,800	Primigravid n = 42,446
		Medication n = 1,385	Primigravid n = 42,446
		All methods ≥13 weeks n = 431	Primigravid n = 42,446
		All methods <13 weeks n = 2,315	Primigravid n = 42,446
Jackson et al. (2007)	United States (1995–2003)	D&E 12–24 weeks n = 85	Women with no history of midtrimester abortion, matched by age n = 170

NOTES: The term "primigravid" refers to a first pregnancy.
[a]All methods n = 2,497; primigravid n = 33,520.
[b]All methods n = 689; primigravid n = 8,916.
[c]Aspiration n = 1,421; primigravid n = 33,520.
[d]Aspiration n = 367; primigravid n = 8,916.
[e]Medication n = 1,064; primigravid n = 33,520.

	Adjusted Odds Ratios (Confidence Intervals)		
Hypertension	Antepartum Hemorrhage	Postpartum Hemorrhage	Notes
1.07 (0.92–1.24)	n/a	n/a	aOR (95% CI); control variables not reported
0.69 (0.61–0.78)	1.26 (1.10–1.45)	Vaginal delivery[a] 1.14 (0.97–1.33) Cesarean section[b] 1.01 (0.74–1.36)	aOR (99% CI) adjusted for maternal age at delivery, smoking, and social class
0.73 (0.62–0.85)	1.33 (1.11–1.59)	Vaginal delivery[c] 0.88 (0.71–1.11) Cesarean section[d] 0.96 (0.64–1.45)	
0.63 (0.52–0.76)	1.18 (0.95–1.46)	Vaginal delivery[e] 1.49 (1.21–1.85) Cesarean section[f] 1.06 (0.69–1.62)	
0.83 (0.71–0.98)	1.02 (0.84–1.25)	Vaginal delivery[g] 1.05 (0.85–1.29) Cesarean section[h] 0.94 (0.60–1.45)	
0.64 (0.55–0.75)	1.29 (1.10–1.51)	Vaginal delivery[i] 1.09 (0.90–1.31) Cesarean section[j] 0.94 (0.66–1.35)	
n/a	n/a	n/a	Odds ratios not reported; outcomes reported as percentages (abortion versus control) Abnormal placentation: 4.8% versus 2.4% (p = .310) Hemorrhage: 2.3% versus 2.3% (p = 1.0)

[f]Medication n = 321; primigravid n = 8,916.
[g]All methods ≥13 weeks n = 344; primigravid n = 33,520.
[h]All methods ≥13 weeks n = 87; primigravid n = 8,916.
[i]All methods <13 weeks n = 1,818; primigravid n = 33,520.
[j]All methods <13 weeks n = 497; primigravid n = 8,916.

in their first pregnancy (aOR = 0.64; 99% CI = 0.55–0.75 and aOR = 0.83; 99% CI = 0.71–0.98, respectively).

Does Abortion Increase the Risk of Complications of the Placenta?

Abnormal placentation, including placenta previa and accreta, is associated with maternal hemorrhage requiring transfusion (Saleh, 2008). The committee identified one study that assessed the risk of placenta complications in a full-term pregnancy following an abortion. As noted earlier, Jackson and colleagues (2007) compared the pregnancy outcomes of women with and without a prior D&E in two Chicago-area hospitals (Jackson et al., 2007). The authors found no association between D&E and abnormal placentation.

Does Abortion Increase the Risk of Hemorrhage in Subsequent Pregnancy?

Two types of hemorrhaging may occur during pregnancy and childbirth: antepartum and postpartum. Antepartum hemorrhage—bleeding from or into the genital tract—affects from 3 to 5 percent of pregnancies globally (Lange and Toledo, 2017). Its causes vary with weeks' gestation. Before 20 weeks, bleeding may be due to abnormal embryo implantation, miscarriage, ectopic pregnancy, gestational trophoblastic disease, and benign and malignant tumors of the reproductive tract. After 20 weeks' gestation (and before birth), the most common causes of antepartum bleeding are cervical change due to preterm labor and disorders of the placenta. Postpartum hemorrhage is usually defined as the loss of 500 ml or more of blood from the genital tract within 24 hours of childbirth (RCOG, 2017); in 2006, it affected an estimated 2.9 percent of pregnancies in the United States (Callaghan et al., 2010). The most common cause (79 percent) is uterine atony, the failure of the uterus to contract following delivery (Bateman et al., 2010).

The Woolner et al. (2014) registry study contains the only analysis the committee could identify on abortion's association with hemorrhage in subsequent pregnancy (Woolner et al., 2014). The study found that prior aspiration abortion was associated with a higher risk of antepartum hemorrhage (aOR = 1.33; 99% CI = 1.11–1.59). However, unlike the other outcomes the researchers investigated (e.g., see the above review of hypertensive disorders and preterm birth), antepartum hemorrhage was not clearly defined, and the finding of higher risk does not appear to be clinically significant as there was no association with preterm birth or hospitalization. In contrast, Woolner and colleagues (2014) clearly defined postpartum hemorrhage as >500 ml blood loss for vaginal delivery or >1,000 ml blood loss for cesarean section. The risk of postpartum hemorrhage during a vaginal delivery was higher among women who had had a medication abortion (but not an aspiration abortion) compared with women in their first pregnancy (aOR = 1.49; 99% CI = 1.21–1.85). It is unclear how a medication abortion might lead to postpartum hemorrhage in a later pregnancy. There were no differences for cesarean section.

Preterm Birth, Small for Gestational Age, and Low Birthweight

Preterm birth (birth at <37 weeks' gestation) and low birthweight are related. Infants born prematurely are more likely than full-term infants to weigh <2,500 g (the definition of low birthweight)—although full-term infants that are small for gestational age may also weigh <2,500 g, and low-birthweight and preterm infants can be the appropriate weight for their gestation. Each of these adverse outcomes may have different underlying causes. The risks to neonatal survival and development vary at different birthweights and weeks' gestation. Thus, investigators often examine both gestation at delivery and fetal growth to determine whether a prior abortion is a risk factor for poor pregnancy outcomes in the future.

First births are at greater risk of preterm delivery than are subsequent births (Ananth et al., 2001). Thus, if the risk of preterm delivery is compared for women who have had an abortion and those who have not, the findings are likely to be biased if they do not take into account the increased risk of preterm delivery for first births (Hogue et al., 1982). To address this source of bias and ensure the comparability of study populations, the committee limited its review to studies of preterm birth that compare the outcomes of a first birth or control for the number of previous births. In the following discussion, the extent to which studies adjust for other confounding variables (e.g., smoking, maternal age, the provision of prophylactic antibiotics at the time of abortion, the type of abortion method, weeks' gestation, and the number of prior abortions) is noted.

The committee identified five studies that met its criteria for assessing the association of abortion with birth outcomes (see Table 4-2). These include the Woolner et al. (2014) and Jackson et al. (2007) studies described above and three studies that used linked Finnish medical records during different but overlapping time periods (KC et al., 2017b; Klemetti et al., 2012; Mannisto et al., 2017). The findings from these studies are presented below. See Table 4-2 for further details on study designs and results.

Do Early-Gestation Aspiration or Medication Abortions Increase the Risk of Preterm Birth?

The Woolner et al. (2014) study is the only available reliable analysis (meeting the committee's criteria) of the association between abortion

TABLE 4-2 Studies Assessing the Association Between Abortion and Preterm Birth (PTB), Low Birthweight (LBW), and Small for Gestational Age (SGA) Using Record-Linkage Methods

Authors (year)	Location (abortion period)	Abortion Group	Comparator	Adjusted Odds Ratios (Confidence Intervals) Very PTB[a]
KC et al. (2017b)	Finland (1983–2013)	1 medication abortion n = 12,183	No previous abortion n = 365,356	Very PTB 0.92 (0.70–1.21) Extremely PTB 0.96 (0.68–1.35)
		1 aspiration abortion n = 33,840	No previous abortion n = 365,356	Very PTB 1.01 (0.87–1.18) Extremely PTB 1.11 (0.92–1.33)
		>1 medication abortion n = 1,267	No previous abortion n = 365,356	Very PTB 0.50 (0.16–1.55) Extremely PTB 0.82 (0.26–2.58)
		>1 aspiration abortion n = 4,819	No previous abortion n = 365,356	Very PTB 1.14 (0.81–1.59) Extremely PTB 1.51 (1.03–2.23)
Mannisto et al. (2017)	Finland (2000–2009)	0 to <6 months interpregnancy interval n = 2,956	18 to <24 months interpregnancy interval n = 2,076	n/a
		6 to <12 months interpregnancy interval n = 3,203	18 to <24 months interpregnancy interval n = 2,076	n/a
		12 to <18 months interpregnancy interval n = 2,623	18 to <24 months interpregnancy interval n = 2,076	n/a
		≥24 months interpregnancy interval n = 9,036	18 to <24 months interpregnancy interval n = 2,076	n/a

Adjusted Odds Ratios (Confidence Intervals)			
All PTB <37 Weeks	Spontaneous PTB <37 Weeks	LBW or SGA	Notes
0.85 (0.77–0.93)	n/a	SGA 1.05 (0.97–1.15)	aOR (95% CI) adjusted for maternal age, marital status, maternal smoking, maternal residence of municipality, and birth year of child.
0.99 (0.94–1.05)	n/a	SGA 1.07 (1.02–1.13)	
0.70 (0.51–0.96)	n/a	SGA 1.05 (0.82–1.34)	
1.00 (0.88–1.14)	n/a	SGA 1.07 (0.95–1.21)	
1.35 (1.02–1.77)	n/a	LBW 1.22 (0.90–1.66) SGA 1.15 (0.80–1.66)	aOR (95% CI) adjusted for parity, prepregnancy body mass index (BMI), cohabitation, type of residence, socioeconomic status, maternal age, smoking, type of termination of pregnancy, and gestational age at termination of pregnancy.
1.14 (0.86–1.50)	n/a	LBW 1.10 (0.82–1.49) SGA 1.21 (0.85–1.71)	
0.94 (0.70–1.26)	n/a	LBW 0.87 (0.62–1.20) SGA 0.86 (0.58–1.26)	
1.19 (0.93–1.53)	n/a	LBW 1.06 (0.81–1.39) SGA 0.89 (0.65–1.22)	

continued

TABLE 4-2 Continued

Authors (year)	Location (abortion period)	Abortion Group	Comparator	Adjusted Odds Ratios (Confidence Intervals) Very PTB[a]
Woolner et al. (2014)	Scotland (1986–2010)	All methods n = 3,186	No previous pregnancy n = 42,446	0.81 (0.54–1.21)
		Aspiration n = 1,800	No previous pregnancy n = 42,446	0.73 (0.42–1.26)
		Medication n = 1,385	No previous pregnancy n = 42,446	0.91 (0.52–1.60)
		All methods <13 weeks n = 2,315	No previous pregnancy n = 42,446	0.84 (0.53–1.33)
		All methods ≥13 weeks n = 431	No previous pregnancy n = 42,446	1.02 (0.64–1.62)
Klemetti et al. (2012)	Finland (1983–2008)	1 previous abortion n = 31,083	No previous abortion n = 264,190	1.19 (0.98–1.44)
		2 previous abortions n = 4,417	No previous abortion n = 264,190	1.69 (1.14–2.51)
		3 or more previous abortions n = 942	No previous abortion n = 264,190	2.78 (1.48–5.24)
		1 or more previous abortions n = 36,442	No previous abortion n = 264,190	1.27 (1.06–1.52)

Adjusted Odds Ratios (Confidence Intervals)			
All PTB <37 Weeks	Spontaneous PTB <37 Weeks	LBW or SGA	Notes
1.05 (0.88–1.26)	1.05 (0.83–1.32)[b]	LBW 1.14 (0.94–1.39)	aOR (99% CI) adjusted for maternal age at delivery, smoking, and social class.
1.10 (0.88–1.39)	1.06 (0.78–1.44)[c]	LBW 1.08 (0.84–1.38)	
0.98 (0.75–1.29)	1.03 (0.72–1.46)[d]	LBW 1.23 (0.92–1.68)	
1.03 (0.83–1.27)	0.97 (0.73–1.28)[e]	LBW 1.13 (0.90–1.41)	
1.13 (0.91–1.40)	1.25 (0.97–1.60)[f]	LBW 1.01 (0.79–1.29)	
0.98 (0.93–1.03)	n/a	LBW 0.96 (0.90–1.01) Very LBW 1.03 (0.91–1.18)	aOR (95% CI) adjusted for age, marital status, socioeconomic position, urbanity, smoking, miscarriage, and ectopic pregnancy.
1.01 (0.89–1.15)	n/a	LBW 1.02 (0.89–1.18) Very LBW 1.13 (0.84–1.54)	
1.35 (1.07–1.71)	n/a	LBW 1.43 (1.12–1.84) Very LBW 2.25 (1.43–3.52)	
0.99 (0.94–1.04)	n/a	LBW 0.98 (0.93–1.03) Very LBW 1.06 (0.94–1.19)	

continued

TABLE 4-2 Continued

Authors (year)	Location (abortion period)	Abortion Group	Comparator	Adjusted Odds Ratios (Confidence Intervals) Very PTB[a]
Jackson et al. (2007)	United States (1995–2003)	D&E 12–24 weeks n = 85	Women with no history of midtrimester abortion, matched by age n = 170	n/a

NOTES: aOR = adjusted odds radio; CI = confidence interval; LBW = <2,500 g; n/a = not applicable; very LBW = <1,500 g.

[a]Very PTB is defined as the following in these studies: KC et al. (2017b) defines very PTB as a birth before 32 weeks' gestations and extremely PTB as a birth before 28 weeks' gestation; Woolner et al. (2014) defines very PTB as a birth before 33 weeks' gestation; Klemetti et al. (2012) defines very PTB as a birth occurring before 28 weeks' gestation.

[b]All methods n = 2,093; primigravid n = 28,012.

[c]Aspiration n = 1,187; primigravid n = 28,012.

[d]Medication n = 906; primigravid n = 28,012.

[e]All methods <13 weeks n = 1,504; primigravid n = 28,012.

[f]All methods ≥13 weeks n = 304; primigravid n = 28,012.

[g]The authors of this study note that this finding was not likely to be clinically significant and may have been confounded by multiple factors (e.g., an unusually low proportion of PTB in the control group), and that controls were lacking for important variables, including race, socioeconomic status, smoking, and prior uterine surgery (including dilation and curettage) (Jackson et al., 2007, Table 1).

Adjusted Odds Ratios (Confidence Intervals)			
All PTB <37 Weeks	Spontaneous PTB <37 Weeks	LBW or SGA	Notes
n/a	n/a	n/a	Odds ratios not reported; outcomes reported as percentages (abortion versus control): PTB <37 weeks: 9.5% versus 2.9% (p = .025)[g] PTB <34 weeks: 0.0% versus 0.6% (p = 1.0) Spontaneous PTB <37 weeks: 6.0% versus 2.4% (p = .144)

method at ≤13 weeks' gestation and preterm birth in the next pregnancy. As noted above, the authors controlled for smoking history and other potential confounding variables and also stratified the sample to assess differences in the outcomes of women with a prior medication abortion (n = 1,385), a prior aspiration abortion (n = 1,800), or no prior abortion (n = 42,446) both before and after 13 weeks' gestation. The authors found no statistically significant association between an abortion at <13 weeks' gestation in the first pregnancy and preterm (aOR = 1.03; 99% CI = 0.83–1.27), spontaneous preterm (aOR = 0.97; 99% CI = 0.73–1.28), or very preterm births (aOR = 0.84; 99% CI = 0.53–1.33) in the next pregnancy.

Do Later-Gestation Abortions Increase the Risk of Preterm Birth?

Woolner and colleagues (2014) found no significant association between a medication or aspiration abortion after 13 weeks' gestation and a later preterm birth (aOR = 1.13; 99% CI = 0.91–1.40). The small hospital-based study by Jackson and colleagues (2007) compared the birth outcomes of women undergoing D&Es at 12 to 24 weeks' gestation (n = 85) and women without a history of abortion (n = 170). Controlling for maternal age, multiparity, prior preterm birth, first-trimester dilation and curettage, first-trimester spontaneous delivery, and prior cervical surgery, the researchers found no significant difference in the risk of a later spontaneous preterm birth between the groups of women with a prior D&E abortion and no prior abortion.

Does a Short Interval Between Abortion and Subsequent Pregnancy Increase the Risk of Preterm Birth?

A number of studies indicate that a short interpregnancy interval between live births (conception less than 6 months after the previous pregnancy) may be a risk factor for preterm birth (Smith et al., 2003; Wong et al., 2016). Pregnancies occurring 18 to 23 months after a previous birth have been found to have the lowest risks of preterm births and other adverse events (Ball et al., 2004). The committee identified one study that examined whether a short interpregnancy interval after abortion increases the risk of preterm birth in a subsequent birth. In a Finnish-based study of linked medical records, Mannisto and colleagues (2017) addressed this question by comparing postabortion pregnancies occurring less than 6 months after an abortion with those occurring 18 to 23 months postabortion with respect to risk of preterm birth. They found a slight but significant increase in the estimated risk of preterm birth (aOR = 1.35; 95% CI = 1.02–1.77). This finding is consistent with those from studies focused on other pregnancy outcomes in the index pregnancy (Conde-Agudelo et al., 2012; Shachar et al., 2016; Wendt et al., 2012), although some have challenged whether the association is causal or related to maternal factors rather than the interval itself (Ball et al., 2014; Hanley et al., 2017; Klebanoff, 2017). If the association between short interpregnancy interval and preterm birth is causal, extending the interval between pregnancies beyond 6 months should reduce the risk of preterm birth associated with shorter intervals. In the case of abortion, effective postabortion contraceptive counseling and use could reduce this concern.

Do Multiple Abortions Increase the Risk of Preterm Birth?

The committee identified two studies (both based in Finland) that examined whether having multiple abortions is associated with a greater risk of preterm birth (KC et al., 2017b; Klemetti et al., 2012). Using 1983–2008 national registry data, Klemetti and colleagues (2012) compared the outcomes of first-time births among women with two prior abortions of any type or gestation (n = 4,417), three or more prior abortions (n = 942), and no prior abortion (n = 264,190). Their analysis adjusted for maternal age, marital status, socioeconomic status, urban residence, smoking, miscarriage, and ectopic pregnancy. The researchers found a dose-response relationship between the number of prior abortions before a first birth and an increased risk of *very* preterm birth (<28 weeks' gestation)[6] after two abortions (aOR = 1.69; 95% CI = 1.14, 2.51) and after three or more abortions (aOR = 2.78; 95% CI = 1.48, 5.24) compared with first births among women with no abortion history. In addition, three or more abortions were associated with preterm birth at <37 weeks' gestation (aOR = 1.35; 95% CI = 1.07–1.71).

KC and colleagues (2017b)[7] used Finnish registry data that extended into a more recent time period (1983–2013) to examine first-birth outcomes following more than one medication or aspiration abortion. The analysis controlled for maternal age, marital status, smoking, maternal residence (by municipality), and birth year. The researchers found that first births were at an increased risk of very preterm birth[8] after more than one aspiration abortion (n = 4,819) compared with women with no abortions (n = 365,356) (aOR = 1.51; 95% CI = 1.03–2.23). No association was found between multiple medication abortions (n = 1,267) and preterm birth.

---

[6]Incidence of very preterm births (number per 1,000 births): no previous abortions, 3/1,000; one previous abortion, 4/1,000; two previous abortions 6/1,000; three or more previous abortions 11/1,000 (Klemetti et al., 2012).

[7]Another publication by KC and colleagues describes the same study (KC et al., 2017a).

[8]KC and colleagues (2017b) use the term "extremely preterm" to refer to births at <28 weeks. Other than the aORs described, the authors did not report the number of very preterm births in the study groups.

RISK OF BREAST CANCER

Does Abortion Increase the Risk of Breast Cancer?

The association of breast cancer and abortion has been examined in the literature over several decades. Pregnancy has been shown to have a protective effect against breast cancer (NCI, 2016). The original hypotheses suggesting a possible association of abortion with breast cancer drew on animal studies indicating that an *interrupted* pregnancy might reduce the protective effect of full-term pregnancy on future risk of breast cancer (Russo and Russo, 1980). Epidemiological studies have explored this possible association in analyses of women who have had an abortion. However, much of this literature, including systematic reviews, meta-analyses, and primary research, is flawed by recall bias and lack of controls for such clinically important confounding factors as age at first live birth. The risk of hormone receptor-positive breast cancer increases with a woman's age at first full-term pregnancy (NCI, 2016).

The committee identified three case control studies of insured women with abortion coverage that used documented records of a prior abortion (Brewster et al., 2005; Goldacre et al., 2001; Newcomb and Mandelson, 2000). The studies controlled for a variety of confounding variables, such as parity, age at delivery of first child, age at breast cancer diagnosis, family history of breast cancer, race, and socioeconomic status.

In a case control study of Scottish women, Brewster and colleagues (2005) linked National Health Service (NHS) hospital discharge and maternity records with national cancer registry and death records dating from 1981 to 1998. The analysis included 2,833 cases (women with a first-time breast cancer diagnosis before age 55) and 9,888 matched controls (women without cancer who had been admitted to an acute care hospital for a nonobstetric, nongynecological condition). Controls were matched with cases by birth year, year of breast cancer diagnosis, residence, and socioeconomic status. The sample was stratified by the same variables, as well as age at breast cancer diagnosis, parity, and age at delivery of first child. Women who had had a prior abortion were no more likely than other women to develop breast cancer (aOR = 0.80; 95% CI = 0.72–0.89). Age at abortion, number of abortions, weeks of gestation, time since abortion, and temporal sequence of live births and abortions also were not found to increase the risk of breast cancer.

In another case control study using linked NHS records, Goldacre and colleagues (2001) analyzed 28,616 breast cancer cases in the Oxford health region of England from 1968 to 1998. The matched control group included 325,456 women who had been hospitalized for reasons other than cancer. The sample was stratified by age, year of the case or control event, residence, and social class. Women with a prior abortion were found not to be at higher risk of breast cancer than women with no abortion history (OR = 0.83; 95% CI = 0.74–0.93).

Newcomb and Mandelson (2000) analyzed the risk of breast cancer among members of the Group Health Cooperative of Puget Sound (Washington State) by linking health plan and local cancer registry data. The analysis included 138 cancer cases and 252 matched controls and adjusted for race, age at first birth, menopause status, family breast cancer history, and body mass index. The control group was matched by age and period of enrollment in the health plan. The analysis found no association between a history of abortion and breast cancer; compared with women with no prior abortion, the adjusted relative risk of breast cancer in women with an abortion was 0.9 (95% CI = 0.5–1.6).

MENTAL HEALTH DISORDERS

Does Abortion Increase the Risk of Long-Term Mental Health Problems?

The committee identified a wide array of research on mental health outcomes, including systematic reviews (Bellieni and Buonocore, 2013; Charles et al., 2008; Coleman, 2011; Fergusson et al., 2013; Major et al., 2008, 2009; NCCMH, 2011), prospective cohort studies (Biggs et al., 2015, 2016, 2017; Foster et al., 2015; Munk-Olsen et al., 2011), cohort studies (Fergusson et al., 2006; Gomez, 2018; Herd et al., 2016; Pedersen, 2007, 2008; Steinberg and Russo, 2008; Steinberg et al., 2011; Warren et al., 2010), and analyses linking medical record or registry data (Coleman et al., 2002; Gissler et al., 2015; Leppalahti et al., 2016; Munk-Olsen et al., 2011; Reardon et al., 2003). Most of the studies focused on whether abortion increases women's risk of depression, anxiety, and/or posttraumatic stress disorder (PTSD).

The utility of most of the published research on mental health outcomes is limited by selective recall bias, inadequate controls for confounding factors, and inappropriate comparators (Major et al., 2008; NCCMH, 2011). Moreover, systematic reviews and meta-analyses are not reliable if they do not assess the quality of the primary research they include (IOM, 2011). As noted earlier, objective documentation of a prior abortion is essential to assessing whether abortion is associated with any outcomes, including subsequent mental health problems. Yet while self-reported data are not reliable sources of abortion history, self-reports are the basis of much of the available primary research on the association between abortion and mental health (Fergusson et al., 2006; Gomez, 2018; Herd et al., 2016; Nilsen et al., 2012; Pedersen, 2007, 2008; Steinberg and Finer, 2011; Steinberg and Russo, 2008; Steinberg et al., 2011; Sullins, 2016; Warren et al., 2010). In addition, as noted earlier, if a study's objective is to determine whether having an abortion raises the risk of future mental health problems, it is important that the study control for women's mental health status at baseline (i.e., before they had the abortion). For example, Steinberg and colleagues (2014) found that women who have abortions report higher rates of mood disorders (depression, bipolar disorder, and dysthymia) (21.0 percent) before undergoing the procedure compared with women with no abortion history who give birth (10.6 percent). Studies by Coleman and colleagues (2002) and Reardon and colleagues (2003) failed to control adequately for preexisting mental disorders. Munk-Olsen and colleagues (2011, 2012) report that their analyses are limited because they were unable to control for a woman's reason for having an abortion and whether the pregnancy was unwanted. Terminations of pregnancies due to fetal abnormalities, for example, may have very different psychological consequences than abortions for unwanted pregnancies.[9]

The committee identified seven systematic reviews on the association between abortion and long-term mental health problems (Bellieni and Buonocore, 2013; Charles et al., 2008; Coleman, 2011; Fergusson et al., 2013; Major et al., 2008, 2009; NCCMH, 2011). The 2011 review conducted by the UK National Collaborating Center for Mental Health (NCCMH)[10] is particularly informative (NCCMH, 2011). Building on the previously published reviews, the NCCMH (2011) used GRADE[11] to analyze the quality of individual studies on several research questions, including the focus of this review, that is, whether women who have an abortion experience more mental health problems than women who deliver an unwanted pregnancy. The two reviews published after the NCCMH report (Bellieni and Buonocore, 2013; Fergusson et al., 2013) identified no additional studies that met the committee's selection criteria. After extensive quality checks of the primary literature, including controlling for previous mental health problems, NCCMH (2011) found that "the rates of mental health problems for women with an unwanted pregnancy were the same whether they had an abortion or gave birth" (p. 8).

The committee identified several more recent studies that met its selection criteria but were published after the NCCMH and other systematic reviews (Biggs et al., 2015, 2016, 2017; Foster et al., 2015; Leppalahti et

---

[9]The committee did not examine the literature on the mental health consequences of terminations of pregnancies due to fetal abnormalities.

[10]The NCCMH was established by the Royal College of Psychiatrists, in partnership with the British Psychological Society, to develop evidence-based mental health reviews and clinical guidelines (NCCMH, 2011).

[11]GRADE refers to the Grading of Recommendations Assessment, Development, and Evaluation. It is a tool, used by the Cochrane Collaboration and many other health care research organizations, for assessing the quality of evidence in health care and the strength of clinical recommendations (GRADE Working Group, 2004, 2018).

al., 2016). Four recent articles draw on the Turnaway study, a prospective longitudinal cohort study designed to address many of the limitations of other studies (Biggs et al., 2015, 2016, 2017; Foster et al., 2015).

The Turnaway study contributes unique insight into the consequences of receiving a desired abortion versus being denied the procedure and carrying the pregnancy to term. The study sample included 956 English- and Spanish-speaking women aged 15 and over who sought abortions between 2008 and 2010 from 30 abortion facilities in the United States. The sample design was unique because it drew from groups of women who presented up to 3 weeks beyond a facility's gestational age limit and were denied an abortion, women presenting within 2 weeks of the limit who received an abortion, and women who received a first-trimester abortion. The women were followed via semiannual phone interviews for 5 years (Dobkin et al., 2014). The investigators collected baseline data on mental health (history of depression, anxiety, suicidal ideation), as well as data on factors known to be important predictors of mental health problems (e.g., history of trauma and abuse). The study groups were specifically designed to enable comparisons of women who had had abortions and those who had been turned away (wanted an abortion but were denied one).

Results from the Turnaway study suggest that there are few psychiatric consequences of abortion, including risk of depression, anxiety, or PTSD. At 2 years, women who had received an abortion had similar or lower levels of depression and anxiety than women denied an abortion (Foster et al., 2015). The study also examined new self-reports of professional diagnoses of either depression or anxiety at 3 years postabortion. Women who had obtained abortions near facility gestational limits were at no greater mental health risk than women who had sought an abortion and carried an unwanted pregnancy to term (Biggs et al., 2015). At 4 years follow-up, the participants completed a measure of PTSD risk (Biggs et al., 2016). Women who had received an abortion were at no higher risk of PTSD than women who had been denied an abortion. At 5 years follow-up, women completed measures of mental health (depression and anxiety) and well-being (self-esteem and life satisfaction) (Biggs et al., 2017). Compared with having had an abortion, having being denied an abortion may be associated with greater risk of initially experiencing more anxiety symptoms; levels of depression were similar among both groups of women.

Two recent studies used Finnish registry data to analyze mental health outcomes after abortion. Leppalahti and colleagues (2016) conducted a longitudinal retrospective cohort study of girls born in Finland in 1987 to examine the effect of abortion on adolescent girls. The comparison groups were girls who had had an abortion (n = 1,041) or given birth (n = 394) before age 18 and a group with no pregnancies up to age 20 (n = 25,312). The girls were followed until age 25. The researchers found no significant differences between the underage abortion group and childbirth group with respect to risk of any psychiatric disorder (including psychoactive substance use disorder, mood disorder, or neurotic or stress-related disorders) after the index pregnancy (aOR = 0.96; 95% CI = 0.67–1.40). Other recent Finnish research provides some evidence that monitoring for mental health status in a follow-up visit after abortion may help reduce the consequences of serious mental health disorders (Gissler et al., 2015).

PREMATURE DEATH

Does Abortion Increase the Risk of Premature Death?

Mortality following abortion is an important long-term outcome to consider. As noted in Chapter 2 (see Table 2-4), when mortality rates from abortion and childbirth are compared, abortion is associated with fewer maternal deaths than carrying a pregnancy to term (Grimes, 2006; Raymond and Grimes, 2012). However, the follow-up period in these short-term studies may not have been of sufficient length to account for late complications leading to death. The committee identified several studies that examined long-term mortality and abortion. These studies—one U.S. study (Reardon et al., 2002) and four studies using Finnish registries (Gissler et al., 2004, 2005, 2015; Jalanko et al., 2017)—are based on linked records. In comparing groups on mortality, however, it is important to adjust for both individual characteristics and social risk factors, as they are likely to differ between women who give birth and those who have an abortion. Minority women and those who are young, unmarried, or poor are more likely than more advantaged women to have unwanted pregnancies and subsequent abortions (Boonstra et al., 2006). Without robust risk adjustments for these social differences, attributing outcomes to such factors as having an abortion or not, especially when the outcomes are rare, is inappropriate. As a result of the inability to control for the many ways in which women who have unwanted pregnancies differ from those who do not, no clear conclusions regarding the association between abortion and long-term mortality can be drawn from these studies.

SUMMARY

This chapter has reviewed the epidemiological evidence on abortion's long-term effects on future childbearing and pregnancy outcomes, risk of breast cancer, mental health disorders, and premature death. The committee found that much of the published literature on these topics fails to meet scientific standards for rigorous, unbiased research. Reliable research on these outcomes uses documented records of a prior abortion, analyzes comparable study and control groups, and controls for confounding variables shown to affect the outcome of interest. Thus, this chapter has focused on the findings of research that meets these basic standards. The committee did not find well-designed research on abortion's association with future ectopic pregnancy, miscarriage or stillbirth, or long-term mortality. Findings on hemorrhage during a subsequent pregnancy are inconclusive.

The committee identified high-quality research on numerous outcomes of interest and concludes that having an abortion does not increase a woman's risk of secondary infertility, pregnancy-related hypertensive disorders, abnormal placentation (after a D&E abortion), preterm birth, breast cancer, or mental health disorders (depression, anxiety, and PTSD). An increased risk of very preterm birth (<28 weeks' gestation) in a woman's first birth was found to be associated with having two or more prior aspiration abortions compared with first births among women with no abortion history; the risk appears to be associated with the number of prior abortions. Preterm birth is associated with pregnancy spacing after an abortion: it is more likely if the interval between abortion and conception is less than 6 months (the same is also true of pregnancy spacing in general).

REFERENCES

ACOG (American College of Obstetricians and Gynecologists). 2017. *Ectopic pregnancy.* https://www.acog.org/Patients/FAQs/Ectopic-Pregnancy (accessed November 13, 2017).

Alexander, L. K., B. Lopes, K. Ricchetti-Masterson, and K. B. Yeatts. 2015. *ERIC notebook. sources of systematic error or bias: Information bias,* 2nd ed. https://sph.unc.edu/files/2015/07/nciph_ERIC14.pdf (accessed December 4, 2017).

Ananth, C. V., D. P. Misra, K. Demissie, and J. C. Smulian. 2001. Rates of preterm delivery among black women and white women in the United States over two decades: An age-period-cohort analysis. *American Journal of Epidemiology* 154(7):657–665.

Anderson, B. A., K. Katus, A. Puur, and B. D. Silver. 1994. The validity of survey responses on abortion: Evidence from Estonia. *Demography* 31(1):115–132.

Ball, S. J., G. Pereira, P. Jacoby, N. de Klerk, and F. J. Stanley. 2014. Re-evaluation of link between interpregnancy interval and adverse birth outcomes: Retrospective cohort study matching two intervals per mother. *British Medical Journal* 349:g4333. doi:10.1136/bmj.g4333.

Bateman B. T., M. F. Berman, L. E. Riley, and L. R. Leffert. 2010. The epidemiology of postpartum hemorrhage in a large, nationwide sample of deliveries. *Anesthesia-Analgesia* 110(5):1368–1373.

Bellieni, C. V., and G. Buonocore. 2013. Abortion and subsequent mental health: Review of the literature. *Psychiatry and Clinical Neurosciences* 67(5):301–310.

Beral, V., D. Bull, R. Doll, R. Peto, and G. Reeves. 2004. Breast cancer and abortion: Collaborative reanalysis of data from 53 epidemiological studies, including 83,000 women with breast cancer from 16 countries. *Lancet* 363(9414):1007–1016.

Biggs, M. A., J. M. Neuhaus, and D. G. Foster. 2015. Mental health diagnoses 3 years after receiving or being denied an abortion in the United States. *American Journal of Public Health* 105(12):2557–2563.

Biggs, M. A., B. Rowland, C. E. McCulloch, and D. G. Foster. 2016. Does abortion increase women's risk for post-traumatic stress? Findings from a prospective longitudinal cohort study. *British Medical Journal Open* 6(2):e009698. doi:10.1136/bmjopen-2015-009698.

Biggs, M. A., U. D. Upadhyay, C. E. McCulloch, and D. G. Foster. 2017. Women's mental health and well-being 5 years after receiving or being denied an abortion: A prospective, longitudinal cohort study. *JAMA Psychiatry* 74(2):169–178.

Boonstra, H. D., R. Gold, C. Richards, and L. Finer. 2006. *Abortion in women's lives.* New York: Guttmacher Institute.

Bouyer, J., J. Coste, T. Shojaei, J. L. Pouly, H. Fernandez, L. Gerbaud, and N. Job-Spira. 2003. Risk factors for ectopic pregnancy: A comprehensive analysis based on a large case-control, population-based study in France. *American Journal of Epidemiology* 157(3):185–194.

Brewster, D., D. Stockton, R. Dobbie, D. Bull, and V. Beral. 2005. Risk of breast cancer after miscarriage or induced abortion: A Scottish record linkage case-control study. *Journal of Epidemiology and Community Health* 59(4):283–287.

Callaghan, W. M., E. V. Kuklina, and C. J. Berg. 2010. Trends in postpartum hemorrhage: United States, 1994–2006. *American Journal of Obstetrics and Gynecology* 202(4):353, e351–e356.

CDC (Centers for Disease Control and Prevention). 2016. *Pregnancy complications.* https://www.cdc.gov/reproductivehealth/maternalinfanthealth/pregcomplications.htm (accessed February 2, 2018).

Charles, V. E., C. B. Polis, S. K. Sridhara, and R. W. Blum. 2008. Abortion and long-term mental health outcomes: A systematic review of the evidence. *Contraception* 78(6):436–450.

Cochrane Collaboration. 2018. *Assessing risk of bias in included studies.* http://methods.cochrane.org/bias/assessing-risk-bias-included-studies (accessed January 5, 2018).

Coleman, P. K. 2011. Abortion and mental health: Quantitative synthesis and analysis of research published 1995–2009. *The British Journal of Psychiatry* 199(3):180–186.

Coleman, P. K., D. C. Reardon, V. M. Rue, and J. Cougle. 2002. State-funded abortions versus deliveries: A comparison of outpatient mental health claims over 4 years. *American Journal of Orthopsychiatry* 72(1):141–152.

Conde-Agudelo, A., A. Rosas-Bermudez, F. Castano, and M. H. Norton. 2012. Effects of birth spacing on maternal, perinatal, infant, and child health: A systematic review of causal mechanisms. *Studies in Family Planning* 43(2):93–114.

Dobkin, L. M., H. Gould, R. E. Barar, M. Ferrari, E. I. Weiss, and D. G. Foster. 2014. Implementing a prospective study of women seeking abortion in the United States: Understanding and overcoming barriers to recruitment. *Women's Health Issues* 24(1):e115–e123.

Fergusson, D. M., L. J. Horwood, and E. M. Ridder. 2006. Abortion in young women and subsequent mental health. *Journal of Child Psychology and Psychiatry* 47(1):16–24.

Fergusson, D. M., L. J. Horwood, and J. M. Boden. 2013. Does abortion reduce the mental health risks of unwanted or unintended pregnancy? A re-appraisal of the evidence. *Australian & New Zealand Journal of Psychiatry* 47(9):819–827.

Foster, D. G., J. R. Steinberg, S. C. Roberts, J. Neuhaus, and M. A. Biggs. 2015. A comparison of depression and anxiety symptom trajectories between women who had an abortion and women denied one. *Psychological Medicine* 45(10):2073–2082.

Garovic, V. D., and P. August. 2013. Preeclampsia and the future risk of hypertension: The pregnant evidence. *Current Hypertension Reports* 15(2). doi:10.1007/s11906-013-0329-4.

Gissler, M., C. Berg, M.-H. Bouvier-Colle, and P. Buekens. 2004. Pregnancy-associated mortality after birth, spontaneous abortion, or induced abortion in Finland, 1987–2000. *American Journal of Obstetrics and Gynecology* 190(2):422–427.

Gissler, M., C. Berg, M.-H. Bouvier-Colle, and P. Buekens. 2005. Injury deaths, suicides and homicides associated with pregnancy, Finland 1987–2000. *The European Journal of Public Health* 15(5):459–463.

Gissler, M., E. Karalis, and V. M. Ulander. 2015. Decreased suicide rate after induced abortion, after the current care guidelines in Finland 1987–2012. *Scandinavian Journal of Public Health* 43(1):99–101.

Goldacre, M., L. Kurina, V. Seagroatt, and D. Yeates. 2001. Abortion and breast cancer: A case-control record linkage study. *Journal of Epidemiology and Community Health* 55(5):336–337.

Gomez, A. M. 2018. Abortion and subsequent depressive symptoms: An analysis of the National Longitudinal Study of Adolescent Health. *Psychology Medicine* 48(2):294–304. doi:10.1017/S0033291717001684.

GRADE (Grading of Recommendations Assessment, Development and Evaluation) Working Group. 2004. Grading quality of evidence and strength of recommendations. *British Medical Journal* 328(7454):1490.

GRADE Working Group. 2018. *GRADE.* http://www.gradeworkinggroup.org (accessed January 19, 2018).

Grimes, D. A. 2006. Estimation of pregnancy-related mortality risk by pregnancy outcome, United States, 1991 to 1999. *American Journal of Obstetrics and Gynecology* 194(1):92–94.

Hanley, G. E., J. A. Hutcheon, B. A. Kinniburgh, and L. Lee. 2017. Interpregnancy interval and adverse pregnancy outcomes: An analysis of successive pregnancies. *Obstetrics & Gynecology* 129(3):408–415.

Herd, P., J. Higgins, K. Sicinski, and I. Merkurieva. 2016. The implications of unintended pregnancies for mental health in later life. *American Journal of Public Health* 106(3):421–429.

Hogue, C. J. 1975. Low birth weight subsequent to induced abortion. A historical prospective study of 948 women in Skopje, Yugoslavia. *American Journal of Obstetrics and Gynecology* 123(7):675–681.

Hogue, C. J., W. Cates, Jr., and C. Tietze. 1982. The effects of induced abortion on subsequent reproduction. *Epidemiologic Reviews* 4(1):66–94.

Holmlund, S., T. Kauko, J. Matomaki, M. Tuominen, J. Makinen, and P. Rautava. 2016. Induced abortion—impact on a subsequent pregnancy in first-time mothers: A registry-based study. *BMC Pregnancy and Childbirth* 16(1):325.

IOM (Institute of Medicine). 2011. *Finding what works in health care: Standards for systematic reviews.* Washington, DC: The National Academies Press.

Jackson, J. E., W. A. Grobman, E. Haney, and H. Casele. 2007. Mid-trimester dilation and evacuation with laminaria does not increase the risk for severe subsequent pregnancy complications. *International Journal of Gynaecology & Obstetrics* 96(1):12–15.

Jalanko, E., S. Leppalahti, O. Heikinheimo, and M. Gissler. 2017. Increased risk of premature death following teenage abortion and childbirth: A longitudinal cohort study. *European Journal of Public Health* 5(1):845–849.

Jones, R. K., and K. Kost. 2007. Underreporting of induced and spontaneous abortion in the United States: An analysis of the 2002 National Survey of Family Growth. *Studies in Family Planning* 38(3):187–197.

KC, S., E. Hemminki, M. Gissler, S. M. Virtanen, and R. Klemetti. 2017a. Perinatal outcomes after induced termination of pregnancy by methods: A nationwide register-based study of first births in Finland 1996–2013. *PLoS One* 12(9):e0184078. doi: 10.1371/journal.pone.0184078.

KC, S., M. Gissler, S. M. Virtanen, and R. Klemetti. 2017b. Risks of adverse perinatal outcomes after repeat terminations of pregnancy by their methods: A nationwide register-based cohort study in Finland 1996–2013. *Paediatrics and Perinatal Epidemiology* 31(6):485–492.

Klebanoff, M. A. 2017. Interpregnancy interval and pregnancy outcomes: Causal or not? *Obstetrics & Gynecology* 129(3):405–407.

Klemetti, R., M. Gissler, M. Niinimaki, and E. Hemminki. 2012. Birth outcomes after induced abortion: A nationwide register-based study of first births in Finland. *Human Reproduction* 27(11):3315–3320.

Lange, E. M. S., and P. Toledo. 2017. Chapter 33. Antepartum hemorrhage. In *Complications in anesthesia*, 3rd ed., edited by L. A. Fleisher and S. H. Rosenbaum. Philadelphia, PA: W. B. Elsevier.

Leppalahti, S., O. Heikinheimo, I. Kalliala, P. Santalahti, and M. Gissler. 2016. Is underage abortion associated with adverse outcomes in early adulthood? A longitudinal birth cohort study up to 25 years of age. *Human Reproduction* 31(9):2142–2149.

Lindefors-Harris, B. M., G. Eklund, H. O. Adami, and O. Meirik. 1991. Response bias in a case-control study: Analysis utilizing comparative data concerning legal abortions from two independent Swedish studies. *American Journal of Epidemiology* 134(9):1003–1008.

Lowit, A., S. Bhattacharya, and S. Bhattacharya. 2010. Obstetric performance following an induced abortion. *Best Practice & Research in Clinical Obstetrics & Gynaecology* 24(5):667–682.

Major, B., M. Appelbaum, L. Beckman, M. A. Dutton, N. F. Russo, and C. West. 2008. *Report of the APA Task Force on Mental Health and Abortion.* Washington, DC: American Psychological Association.

Major, B., M. Appelbaum, L. Beckman, M. A. Dutton, N. F. Russo, and C. West. 2009. Abortion and mental health: Evaluating the evidence. *American Psychologist* 64(9):863–890.

Mannisto, J., A. Bloigu, M. Mentula, M. Gissler, O. Heikinheimo, and M. Niinimaki. 2017. Interpregnancy interval after termination of pregnancy and the risks of adverse outcomes in subsequent birth. *Obstetrics & Gynecology* 129(2):347–354.

Munk-Olsen, T., T. M. Laursen, C. B. Pedersen, Ø. Lidegaard, and P. B. Mortensen. 2011. Induced first-trimester abortion and risk of mental disorder. *New England Journal of Medicine* 364(4):332–339.

Munk-Olsen, T., T. M. Laursen, C. B. Pedersen, Ø. Lidegaard, and P. B. Mortensen. 2012. First-time first-trimester induced abortion and risk of readmission to a psychiatric hospital in women with a history of treated mental disorder. *Archives of General Psychiatry* 69(2):159–165.

NAF (National Abortion Federation). 2017. *2017 Clinical policy guidelines for abortion care.* Washington, DC: NAF.

NCCMH (National Collaborating Centre for Mental Health). 2011. *Induced abortion and mental health: A systematic review of the mental health outcomes of induced abortion, including their prevalence and associated factors.* London, UK: Academy of Medical Royal Colleges.

NCI (National Cancer Institute). 2016. *Reproductive history and cancer risk.* https://www.cancer.gov/about-cancer/causes-prevention/risk/hormones/reproductive-history-fact-sheet (accessed January 31, 2018).

Newcomb, P. A., and M. T. Mandelson. 2000. A record-based evaluation of induced abortion and breast cancer risk (United States). *Cancer Causes Control* 11(9):777–781.

Nilsen, W., C. A. Olsson, E. Karevold, C. O'Loughlin, M. McKenzie, and G. C. Patton. 2012. Adolescent depressive symptoms and subsequent pregnancy, pregnancy completion and pregnancy termination in young adulthood: Findings from the Victorian Adolescent Health Cohort Study. *Journal of Pediatric and Adolescent Gynecology* 25(1):6–11.

ODPHP (Office of Disease Prevention and Health Promotion). 2017. *National Vital Statistics System—fetal death.* https://www.healthypeople.gov/2020/data-source/national-vital-statistics-system-fetal-death (accessed November 10, 2017).

Pedersen, W. 2007. Childbirth, abortion and subsequent substance use in young women: A population-based longitudinal study. *Addiction* 102(12):1971–1978.

Pedersen, W. 2008. Abortion and depression: A population-based longitudinal study of young women. *Scandinavian Journal of Social Medicine* 36(4):424–428.

Raymond, E. G., and D. A. Grimes. 2012. The comparative safety of legal induced abortion and childbirth in the United States. *Obstetrics & Gynecology* 119(2 Pt. 1):215–219.

RCOG (Royal College of Obstetricians and Gynaecologists). 2011. *The care of women requesting induced abortion* (Evidence-based clinical guideline number 7). https://www.rcog.org.uk/globalassets/documents/guidelines/abortion-guideline_web_1.pdf (accessed July 27, 2017).

RCOG. 2015. *Best practice in comprehensive abortion care* (Best practice paper no. 2). London, UK: RCOG.

RCOG. 2017. Prevention and management of postpartum haemorrhage. *British Journal of Obstetrics & Gynaecology* 124(5):e106–e149.

Reardon, D., J. Cougle, P. Ney, F. Scheuren, P. Coleman, and T. Strahan. 2002. Deaths associated with delivery and abortion among California Medicaid patients: A record linkage study. *The Southern Medical Journal* 95(8):834–841.

Reardon, D. C., J. R. Cougle, V. M. Rue, M. W. Shuping, P. K. Coleman, and P. G. Ney. 2003. Psychiatric admissions of low-income women following abortion and childbirth. *Canadian Medical Association Journal* 168(10):1253–1256.

Roblin, P. 2014. Vacuum aspiration. In *Abortion care*, edited by S. Rowlands. Cambridge, UK: Cambridge University Press.

Russo, J., and I. H. Russo. 1980. Susceptibility of the mammary gland to carcinogenesis. II. Pregnancy interruption as a risk factor in tumor incidence. *American Journal of Pathology* 100(2):497–512.

Saleh, H. 2008. *Placenta previa and accreta.* https://www.glowm.com/section_view/heading/Placenta%20Previa%20and%20Accreta/item/121 (accessed November 13, 2017).

SFP (Society of Family Planning). 2013. Surgical abortion prior to 7 weeks of gestation. *Contraception* 88(1):7–17.

Shachar, B. Z., J. A. Mayo, D. J. Lyell, R. J. Baer, L. L. Jeliffe-Pawlowski, D. K. Stevenson, and G. M. Shaw. 2016. Interpregnancy interval after live birth or pregnancy termination and estimated risk of preterm birth: A retrospective cohort study. *British Journal of Obstetrics & Gynaecology* 123(12):2009–2017.

Sivalingam, V. N., W. C. Duncan, E. Kirk, L. A. Shephard, and A. W. Horne. 2011. Diagnosis and management of ectopic pregnancy. *The Journal of Family Planning and Reproductive Health Care* 37(4):231–240.

Smith, G. C. S., J. P. Pell, and R. Dobbie. 2003. Interpregnancy interval and risk of preterm birth and neonatal death: Retrospective cohort study. *British Medical Journal* 327(7410):313.

Steinberg, J. R., and L. B. Finer. 2011. Examining the association of abortion history and current mental health: A reanalysis of the national comorbidity survey using a common-risk-factors model. *Social Science and Medicine* 72(1):72–82.

Steinberg, J. R., and N. F. Russo. 2008. Abortion and anxiety: What's the relationship? *Social Science & Medicine* 67(2):238–252.

Steinberg, J. R., D. Becker, and J. T. Henderson. 2011. Does the outcome of a first pregnancy predict depression, suicidal ideation, or lower self-esteem? Data from the National Comorbidity Survey. *American Journal of Orthopsychiatry* 81(2):193–201.

Steinberg, J. R., C. E. McCulloch, and N. E. Adler. 2014. Abortion and mental health: Findings from the National Comorbidity Survey-Replication. *Obstetrics & Gynecology* 123(2 Pt. 1):263–270.

Sullins, D. P. 2016. Abortion, substance abuse and mental health in early adulthood: Thirteen-year longitudinal evidence from the United States. *SAGE Open Medicine* 4:2050312116665997.

Tao, G., C. Patel, and K. W. Hoover. 2017. Updated estimates of ectopic pregnancy among commercially and Medicaid-insured women in the United States, 2002–2013. *Southern Medical Journal* 110(1):18–24. doi:10.14423/SMJ.0000000000000594.

Thorp, Jr., J. M., K. E. Hartmann, and E. Shadigian. 2003. Long-term physical and psychological health consequences of induced abortion: Review of the evidence. *Obstetrical & Gynecological Survey* 58(1):67–79.

Warren, J. T., S. M. Harvey, and J. T. Henderson. 2010. Do depression and low self-esteem follow abortion among adolescents? Evidence from a national study. *Perspectives on Sexual and Reproductive Health* 42(4):230–235.

Wendt, A., C. M. Gibbs, S. Peters, and C. J. Hogue. 2012. Impact of increasing inter-pregnancy interval on maternal and infant health. *Paediatric and Perinatal Epidemiology* 26(Suppl. 1):239–258.

WHO (World Health Organization). 2012. *Safe abortion: Technical and policy guidance for health systems*, 2nd ed. http://apps.who.int/iris/bitstream/10665/70914/1/9789241548434_eng.pdf (accessed September 12, 2017).

Wong, L. F., J. Wilkes, K. Korgenski, M. W. Varner, and T. A. Manuck. 2016. Risk factors associated with preterm birth after a prior term delivery. *British Journal of Obstetrics & Gynaecology* 123(11):1772–1778.

Woolner, A., S. Bhattacharya, and S. Bhattacharya. 2014. The effect of method and gestational age at termination of pregnancy on future obstetric and perinatal outcomes: A register-based cohort study in Aberdeen, Scotland. *British Journal of Obstetrics & Gynaecology* 121(3):309–318.

Zhou, W., G. L. Nielsen, H. Larsen, and J. Olsen. 2001. Induced abortion and placenta complications in the subsequent pregnancy. *Acta Obstetricia et Gynecologica Scandinavica* 80(12):1115–1120.

5

Conclusions

This report provides a comprehensive review of the state of the science on the safety and quality of abortion services in the United States. The committee was charged with answering eight specific research questions. This chapter presents the committee's conclusions by responding individually to each question. The research findings that are the basis for these conclusions are presented in the previous chapters. The committee was also asked to offer recommendations regarding the eight questions. However, the committee decided that its conclusions regarding the safety and quality of U.S. abortion care responded comprehensively to the scope of this study. Therefore, the committee does not offer recommendations for specific actions to be taken by policy makers, health care providers, and others.

1. *What types of legal abortion services are available in the United States? What is the evidence regarding which services are appropriate under different clinical circumstances (e.g., based on patient medical conditions such as previous cesarean section, obesity, gestational age)?*

Four legal abortion methods—medication,[1] aspiration, dilation and evacuation (D&E), and induction—are used in the United States. Length of gestation—measured as the amount of time since the first day of the last

---

[1]The terms "medication abortion" and "medical abortion" are used interchangeably in the literature. This report uses "medication abortion" to describe the U.S. Food and Drug Administration (FDA)-approved prescription drug regimen used up to 10 weeks' gestation.

menstrual period—is the primary factor in deciding what abortion procedure is the most appropriate. Both medication and aspiration abortions are used up to 10 weeks' gestation. Aspiration procedures may be used up to 14 to 16 weeks' gestation.

Mifepristone, sold under the brand name Mifeprex, is the only medication specifically approved by the FDA for use in medication abortion. The drug's distribution has been restricted under the requirements of the FDA Risk Evaluation and Mitigation Strategy program since 2011—it may be dispensed only to patients in clinics, hospitals, or medical offices under the supervision of a certified prescriber. To become a certified prescriber, eligible clinicians must register with the drug's distributor, Danco Laboratories, and meet certain requirements. Retail pharmacies are prohibited from distributing the drug.

When abortion by aspiration is no longer feasible, D&E and induction methods are used. D&E is the superior method; in comparison, inductions are more painful for women, take significantly more time, and are more costly. However, D&Es are not always available to women. The procedure is illegal in Mississippi[2] and West Virginia[3] (both states allow exceptions in cases of life endangerment or severe physical health risk to the woman). Elsewhere, access to the procedure is limited because many obstetrician/gynecologists (OB/GYNs) and other physicians lack the requisite training to perform D&Es. Physicians' access to D&E training is very limited or nonexistent in many areas of the country.

Few women are medically ineligible for abortion. There are, however, specific contraindications to using mifepristone for a medication abortion or induction. The drug should not be used for women with confirmed or suspected ectopic pregnancy or undiagnosed adnexal mass; an intrauterine device in place; chronic adrenal failure; concurrent long-term systemic corticosteroid therapy; hemorrhagic disorders or concurrent anticoagulant therapy; allergy to mifepristone, misoprostol, or other prostaglandins; or inherited porphyrias.

Obesity is not a risk factor for women who undergo medication or aspiration abortions (including with the use of moderate intravenous sedation). Research on the association between obesity and complications during a D&E abortion is less certain—particularly for women with Class III obesity (body mass index ≥40) after 14 weeks' gestation.

A history of a prior cesarean delivery is not a risk factor for women undergoing medication or aspiration abortions, but it may be associated

---

[2]Mississippi Unborn Child Protection from Dismemberment Abortion Act, Mississippi HB 519, Reg. Sess. 2015–2016 (2016).

[3]Unborn Child Protection from Dismemberment Abortion Act, West Virginia SB 10, Reg. Sess. 2015–2016 (2016).

with an increased risk of complications during D&E abortions, particularly for women with multiple cesarean deliveries. Because induction abortions are so rare, it is difficult to determine definitively whether a prior cesarean delivery increases the risk of complications. The available research suggests no association.

2. What is the evidence on the physical and mental health risks of these different abortion interventions?

Abortion has been investigated for its potential long-term effects on future childbearing and pregnancy outcomes, risk of breast cancer, mental health disorders, and premature death. The committee found that much of the published literature on these topics does not meet scientific standards for rigorous, unbiased research. Reliable research uses documented records of a prior abortion, analyzes comparable study and control groups, and controls for confounding variables shown to affect the outcome of interest.

Physical health effects The committee identified high-quality research on numerous outcomes of interest and concludes that having an abortion does not increase a woman's risk of secondary infertility, pregnancy-related hypertensive disorders, abnormal placentation (after a D&E abortion), preterm birth, or breast cancer. Although rare, the risk of very preterm birth (<28 weeks' gestation) in a woman's first birth was found to be associated with having two or more prior aspiration abortions compared with first births among women with no abortion history; the risk appears to be associated with the number of prior abortions. Preterm birth is associated with pregnancy spacing after an abortion: it is more likely if the interval between abortion and conception is less than 6 months (this is also true of pregnancy spacing in general). The committee did not find well-designed research on abortion's association with future ectopic pregnancy, miscarriage or still-birth, or long-term mortality. Findings on hemorrhage during a subsequent pregnancy are inconclusive.

Mental health effects The committee identified a wide array of research on whether abortion increases women's risk of depression, anxiety, and/or posttraumatic stress disorder and concludes that having an abortion does not increase a woman's risk of these mental health disorders.

3. What is the evidence on the safety and quality of medical and surgical abortion care?

Safety The clinical evidence clearly shows that legal abortions in the United States—whether by medication, aspiration, D&E, or induction—are safe and effective. Serious complications are rare. But the risk of a serious complication increases with weeks' gestation. As the number of weeks increases, the invasiveness of the required procedure and the need for deeper levels of sedation also increase.

Quality Health care quality is a multidimensional concept. Six attributes of health care quality—safety, effectiveness, patient-centeredness, timeliness, efficiency, and equity—were central to the committee's review of the quality of abortion care. Table 5-1 details the committee's conclusions regarding each of these quality attributes. Overall, the committee concludes that the quality of abortion care depends to a great extent on where women live. In many parts of the country, state regulations have created barriers to optimizing each dimension of quality care. The quality of care is optimal when the care is based on current evidence and when trained clinicians are available to provide abortion services.

4. *What is the evidence on the minimum characteristics of clinical facilities necessary to effectively and safely provide the different types of abortion interventions?*

Most abortions can be provided safely in office-based settings. No special equipment or emergency arrangements are required for medication abortions. For other abortion methods, the minimum facility characteristics depend on the level of sedation that is used. Aspiration abortions are performed safely in office and clinic settings. If moderate sedation is used, the facility should have emergency resuscitation equipment and an emergency transfer plan, as well as equipment to monitor oxygen saturation, heart rate, and blood pressure. For D&Es that involve deep sedation or general anesthesia, the facility should be similarly equipped and also have equipment to provide general anesthesia and monitor ventilation.

Women with severe systemic disease require special measures if they desire or need deep sedation or general anesthesia. These women require further clinical assessment and should have their abortion in an accredited ambulatory surgery center or hospital.

5. *What is the evidence on what clinical skills are necessary for health care providers to safely perform the various components of abortion care, including pregnancy determination, counseling, gestational age assessment, medication dispensing, procedure performance, patient monitoring, and follow-up assessment and care?*

Required skills All abortion procedures require competent providers skilled in patient preparation (education, counseling, and informed consent);

TABLE 5-1 Does Abortion Care in the United States Meet the Six Attributes of Quality Health Care?

Quality Attribute[a]	Definition	Committee's Conclusions
Safety	Avoiding injuries to patients from the care that is intended to help them.	Legal abortions—whether by medication, aspiration, D&E, or induction—are safe. Serious complications are rare and occur far less frequently than during childbirth. Safety is enhanced when the abortion is performed as early in pregnancy as possible.
Effectiveness[b]	Providing services based on scientific knowledge to all who could benefit and refraining from providing services to those not likely to benefit (avoiding underuse and overuse, respectively).	Legal abortions—whether by medication, aspiration, D&E, or induction—are effective. The likelihood that women will receive the type of abortion services that best meets their needs varies considerably depending on where they live. In many parts of the country, abortion-specific regulations on the site and nature of care, provider type, provider training, and public funding diminish this dimension of quality care. The regulations may limit the number of available providers, misinform women of the risks of the procedures they are considering, overrule women's and clinician's medical decision making, or require medically unnecessary services and delays in care. These include policies that • require office-based settings to meet the structural standards of higher-intensity clinical facilities (e.g., ambulatory surgery centers or hospitals) even for the least invasive abortion methods (medication and aspiration); • prohibit the abortion method that is most effective for a particular clinical circumstance (e.g., D&E); • delay care unnecessarily from a clinical standpoint (e.g., mandatory waiting periods); • prohibit qualified clinicians (family medicine physicians, certified nurse-midwives, nurse practitioners, and physician assistants) from performing abortions; • require the informed consent process to include inaccurate information on abortion's long-term physical and mental health effects; • require individual clinicians to have hospital privileges; • bar publicly funded clinics from providing abortion care to low-income women; or • mandate clinically unnecessary services (e.g., preabortion ultrasound, in-person counseling visit).

continued

TABLE 5-1 Continued

Quality Attribute[a]	Definition	Committee's Conclusions
Patient-Centeredness	Providing care that is respectful of and responsive to individual patient preferences, needs, and values and ensuring that patient values guide all clinical decisions.	Patients' personal circumstances and individual preferences (including preferred abortion method), needs, and values may be disregarded depending on where they live (as noted above). The high state-to-state variability regarding the specifics of abortion care may be difficult for patients to understand and navigate. Patients' ability to be adequately informed in order to make sound medical decisions is impeded when state regulations require that • women be provided inaccurate or misleading information about abortion's potential harms; and • women's preferences for whether they want individualized counseling not be taken into consideration.
Timeliness	Reducing waits and sometimes harmful delays for both those who receive and those who give care.	The timeliness of an abortion depends on a variety of local factors, such as the availability of care, affordability, distance from the provider, and state requirements for an in-person counseling appointment and waiting periods (18 to 72 hours) between counseling and the abortion. • There is some evidence that the logistical challenges of arranging and getting to a second appointment can result in delaying the abortion procedure beyond the mandatory waiting period. • Delays put the patient at greater risk of an adverse event.
Efficiency	Avoiding waste, including waste of equipment, supplies, ideas, and energy.	An extensive body of clinical research has led to important refinements and improvements in the procedures, techniques, and methods for performing abortions. The extent to which abortion care is delivered efficiently depends, in part, on the alignment of state regulations with current evidence on best practices. Regulations that require medically unnecessary equipment, services, and/or additional patient visits increase cost, and thus decrease efficiency.

TABLE 5-1 Continued

Quality Attribute[a]	Definition	Committee's Conclusions
Equity	Providing care that does not vary in quality because of personal characteristics such as gender, ethnicity, geographic location, and socioeconomic status.	State-level abortion regulations are likely to affect women differently based on their geographic location and socioeconomic status. Barriers (lack of insurance coverage, waiting periods, limits on qualified providers, and requirements for multiple appointments) are more burdensome for women who reside far from providers and/or have limited resources. • Women who undergo abortions are disproportionately lower-income compared with other women of similar age: family incomes of 49 percent of them are below the federal poverty level (FPL), and family incomes of 26 percent are 100 to 200 percent of the FPL; 61 percent are women of color. • Seventeen percent of women travel more than 50 miles to obtain an abortion.

[a]These attributes of quality health care were first proposed by the Institute of Medicine's Committee on Quality of Health Care in America in the 2001 report *Crossing the Quality Chasm: A New Health System for the 21st Century.*

[b]Elsewhere in this report, effectiveness refers to the successful completion of the abortion without the need for a follow-up aspiration.

clinical assessment (confirming intrauterine pregnancy, determining gestation, taking a relevant medical history, and physical examination); pain management; identification and management of expected side effects and serious complications; and contraceptive counseling and provision. To provide medication abortions, the clinician should be skilled in all these areas. To provide aspiration abortions, the clinician should also be skilled in the technical aspects of an aspiration procedure. To provide D&E abortions, the clinician needs the relevant surgical expertise and sufficient caseload to maintain the requisite surgical skills. To provide induction abortions, the clinician requires the skills needed for managing labor and delivery.

Clinicians that have the necessary competencies Both trained physicians (OB/GYNs, family medicine physicians, and other physicians) and advanced practice clinicians (APCs) (physician assistants, certified nurse-midwives, and nurse practitioners) can provide medication and aspiration abortions safely and effectively. OB/GYNs, family medicine physicians, and other physicians with appropriate training and experience can perform D&E abortions. Induction abortions can be provided by clinicians (OB/GYNs, family medicine physicians, and certified nurse-midwives) with training in managing labor and delivery.

The extensive body of research documenting the safety of abortion care in the United States reflects the outcomes of abortions provided by thousands of individual clinicians. The use of sedation and anesthesia may require special expertise. If moderate sedation is used, it is essential to have a nurse or other qualified clinical staff—in addition to the person performing the abortion—available to monitor the patient, as is the case for any other medical procedure. Deep sedation and general anesthesia require the expertise of an anesthesiologist or certified registered nurse anesthetist to ensure patient safety.

6. What safeguards are necessary to manage medical emergencies arising from abortion interventions?

The key safeguards—for abortions and all outpatient procedures—are whether the facility has the appropriate equipment, personnel, and emergency transfer plan to address any complications that might occur. No special equipment or emergency arrangements are required for medication abortions; however, clinics should provide a 24-hour clinician-staffed telephone line and have a plan to provide emergency care to patients after hours. If moderate sedation is used during an aspiration abortion, the facility should have emergency resuscitation equipment and an emergency transfer plan, as well as equipment to monitor oxygen saturation, heart rate, and blood pressure. D&Es that involve deep sedation or general anesthesia should be provided in similarly equipped facilities that also have equipment to monitor ventilation.

The committee found no evidence indicating that clinicians that perform abortions require hospital privileges to ensure a safe outcome for the patient. Providers should, however, be able to provide or arrange for patient access or transfer to medical facilities equipped to provide blood transfusions, surgical intervention, and resuscitation, if necessary.

7. What is the evidence on the safe provision of pain management for abortion care?

Nonsteroidal anti-inflammatory drugs (NSAIDs) are recommended to reduce the discomfort of pain and cramping during a medication abortion. Some women still report high levels of pain, and researchers are exploring new ways to provide prophylactic pain management for medication abortion. The pharmaceutical options for pain management during aspiration, D&E, and induction abortions range from local anesthesia, to minimal sedation/anxiolysis, to moderate sedation/analgesia, to deep sedation/

analgesia, to general anesthesia. Along this continuum, the physiological effects of sedation have increasing clinical implications and, depending on the depth of sedation, may require special equipment and personnel to ensure the patient's safety. The greatest risk of using sedative agents is respiratory depression. The vast majority of abortion patients are healthy and medically eligible for all levels of sedation in office-based settings. As noted above (see Questions 4 and 6), if sedation is used, the facility should be appropriately equipped and staffed.

8. *What are the research gaps associated with the provision of safe, high-quality care from pre- to postabortion?*

The committee's overarching task was to assess the safety and quality of abortion care in the United States. As noted in the introduction to this chapter, the committee decided that its findings and conclusions fully respond to this charge. The committee concludes that legal abortions are safe and effective. Safety and quality are optimized when the abortion is performed as early in pregnancy as possible. Quality requires that care be respectful of individual patient preferences, needs, and values so that patient values guide all clinical decisions.

The committee did not identify gaps in research that raise concerns about these conclusions and does not offer recommendations for specific actions to be taken by policy makers, health care providers, and others.

The following are the committee's observations about questions that merit further investigation.

Limitation of Mifepristone distribution   As noted above, mifepristone, sold under the brand name Mifeprex, is the only medication approved by the FDA for use in medication abortion. Extensive clinical research has demonstrated its safety and effectiveness using the FDA-recommended regimen. Furthermore, few women have contraindications to medication abortion. Nevertheless, as noted earlier, the FDA REMS restricts the distribution of mifepristone. Research is needed on how the limited distribution of mifepristone under the REMS process impacts dimensions of quality, including timeliness, patient-centeredness, and equity. In addition, little is known about pharmacist and patient perspectives on pharmacy dispensing of mifepristone and the potential for direct-to-patient models through telemedicine.

Pain management   There is insufficient evidence to identify the optimal approach to minimizing the pain women experience during an aspiration procedure without sedation. Paracervical blocks are effective in decreasing procedural pain, but the administration of the block itself is painful, and even with the block, women report experiencing moderate to significant pain. More research is needed to learn how best to reduce the pain women experience during abortion procedures.

Research on prophylactic pain management for women undergoing medication abortions is also needed. Although NSAIDs reduce the pain of cramping, women still report high levels of pain.

Availability of providers   APCs can provide medication and aspiration abortions safely and effectively, but the committee did not find research assessing whether APCs can also be trained to perform D&Es.

Addressing the needs of women of lower income   Women who have abortions are disproportionately poor and at risk for interpersonal and other types of violence. Yet little is known about the extent to which they receive needed social and psychological supports when seeking abortion care or how best to meet those needs. More research is needed to assess the need for support services and to define best clinical practice for providing those services.

Appendix A

Biographical Sketches of
Committee Members

B. Ned Calonge, M.D., M.P.H. (*Co-Chair*), is president and CEO of The Colorado Trust, a private foundation dedicated to achieving health equity for all Coloradans. Prior to joining the Trust, he served as chief medical officer of the Colorado Department of Public Health and Environment. Dr. Calonge also served as chief of the Department of Preventive Medicine for the Colorado Permanente Medical Group (CPMG) and as a CPMG family physician for 10 years. His current academic appointments include associate professor of family medicine, Department of Family Medicine, University of Colorado Denver (UCD) School of Medicine, and associate professor of epidemiology, UCD Colorado School of Public Health. Nationally, Dr. Calonge is past chair of the United States Preventive Services Task Force and a member of the Centers for Disease Control and Prevention's (CDC's) Task Force on Community Preventive Services, as well as the CDC's Breast and Cervical Cancer Early Detection and Control Advisory Committee. He is a past member and chair of the CDC's Evaluating Genomic Applications for Practice and Prevention Workgroup, and is a consultant for and past member of the Advisory Committee on Heritable Disorders in Newborns and Children in the Maternal and Child Health Bureau, Health Resources and Services Administration. Dr. Calonge serves on the Board on Population Health and Public Health Practice and the Roundtable on the Promotion of Health Equity in the Health and Medicine Division of the National Academies of Sciences, Engineering, and Medicine. He has been board-certified in both family medicine and preventive medicine, and was elected to the National Academy of Medicine in 2011. He earned an M.P.H. from the University of Washington and an M.D. from the University of Colorado.

Helene D. Gayle, M.D., M.P.H. (*Co-Chair*), is president and CEO of the Chicago Community Trust. Before assuming leadership of the Trust in October 2017, she served as CEO of McKinsey Social Initiative, a non-profit organization that implements programs that bring together varied stakeholders to address complex global social challenges. A member of the National Academy of Medicine, Dr. Gayle was previously president and CEO of CARE USA, a leading international humanitarian organization with approximately 10,000 staff, whose poverty-fighting programs reached more than 97 million people in 87 countries. An expert on global development, humanitarianism, and health issues, she also spent 20 years with the CDC, focused primarily on combating HIV/AIDS. She was appointed as the first director of the National Center for HIV, STD and TB Prevention, and achieved the rank of rear admiral and assistant surgeon general in the U.S. Public Health Service. Dr. Gayle also served as AIDS coordinator and chief of the HIV/AIDS division for the U.S. Agency for International Development. She then directed the HIV, TB and Reproductive Health Program at the Bill & Melinda Gates Foundation, directing programs on HIV/AIDS and other global health issues. She earned her M.D. at the University of Pennsylvania and an M.P.H. at Johns Hopkins University. She is board-certified in pediatrics.

Wendy R. Brewster, M.D., Ph.D., is a professor and gynecologic oncologist in the Department of Obstetrics and Gynecology and an adjunct professor of epidemiology at the University of North Carolina (UNC) at Chapel Hill. She is also director of the UNC Center for Women's Health Research. Dr. Brewster is a co-investigator for several projects designed to identify populations at risk for disparate treatment and poor outcomes in endometrial, colon, ovarian, and cervical cancers. Her recent work has focused on the paradigm for treatment of gynecologic malignancies where obstacles to treatment exist for high-risk groups in limited-resource areas. Prior to her move to UNC, Dr. Brewster was faculty at the University of California, Irvine. She received her M.D. and completed her residency in obstetrics and gynecology at the University of California, Los Angeles. She completed a fellowship in gynecologic oncology and earned a Ph.D. in environmental analysis and design at the University of California, Irvine. She is board-certified in obstetrics and gynecology and gynecologic oncology.

Lee A. Fleisher, M.D., is currently professor and chair of anesthesiology at the University of Pennsylvania Perelman School of Medicine. His research includes perioperative risk assessment, perioperative quality metrics, and risk adjustment modeling to assess quality of care. He has been involved as a member and chair of professional society guidelines committees and funded by both the Agency for Healthcare Research and Quality and societies to perform evidence-based reviews. Dr. Fleisher was elected to the National Academy of Medicine in 2007. He has been involved in developing performance metrics for both the American Society of Anesthesiologists and the American College of Cardiology. He was chair and is currently a member of the Consensus Standards Advisory Committee and co-chair of the Surgery Standing Committee of the National Quality Forum, and was a member of the Administrative Board of the Council of Faculty and Academic Specialties of the Association of American Medical Colleges. He is also a member of the Medical Advisory Panel of the Technology Evaluation Center of the Blue Cross/Blue Shield Association. He received his M.D. from the State University of New York at Stony Brook, from which he received the Distinguished Alumni Award.

Carol J. Rowland Hogue, Ph.D., M.P.H., is professor of epidemiology and Jules and Uldeen Terry professor of maternal and child health (MCH) at the Rollins School of Public Health, Emory University. She is also director of the Women's and Children's Center and the Health Resources and Services Administration-sponsored Center of Excellence in MCH Education, Science, and Practice. A former director of the federal CDC's Division of Reproductive Health (1988–1992) and on faculties in biometry at the University of Arkansas for Medical Science (1977–1982) and the UNC School of Public Health's Department of Biostatistics (1974–1977), Dr. Hogue initiated many of the current CDC reproductive health programs, including the Pregnancy Risk Assessment Monitoring System, the National Pregnancy Mortality Surveillance System, and the National Infant Mortality Surveillance project, that launched the national- and state-level development and use of linked birth and death records. In addition, she led the first research on maternal morbidities—the precursor to the current safe motherhood initiative—and the initial innovative research on racial disparities in preterm delivery. She has published broadly in maternal health, including studies of long-term complications of induced abortion, ectopic pregnancy, stillbirth, unintended pregnancy, contraceptive failure, and reproductive cancers. Her current research projects include the Stillbirth Collaborative Research Network's population-based case control study of stillbirth, an implementation fidelity study of elementary school-based health centers, and a CDC-sponsored study of the life-course health of adolescents and adults living with congenital heart defects. Among her many honors, Dr. Hogue served as president of the Society for Epidemiologic Research (1988–1989), served on the Institute of Medicine Committee on Unintended Pregnancy (1993–1995), was chair of the Regional Advisory Panel for the Americas of the World Health Organization's Human Reproduction Programme (1997–1999), was president of the American College of Epidemiology (2002–2004), was senior fellow of the Emory Center for the Study of Law and Religion (2001–2006), and received the MCH Coalition's National Effective Practice Award in 2002 and Greg Alexander Award for Advancing Knowledge in 2016. In 2017 she received Emory University's Thomas Jefferson Award, the highest honor awarded to a faculty member.

Jody Rae Lori, Ph.D., R.N., C.N.M., is an associate professor and associate dean for Global Affairs at the University of Michigan School of Nursing (UMSN). She also serves as director of the Pan American Health Organization/World Health Organization Collaborating Center for Nursing and Midwifery at UMSN. A fellow in the American College of Nurse Midwives and the American Academy of Nursing, Dr. Lori focuses her research on the development and testing of new models of care to address the high rates of maternal and neonatal mortality in sub-Saharan Africa. With diverse funding sources, including the National Institutes of Health-Fogarty, the U.S. Agency for International Development, and private foundations, she currently has research projects in Liberia and Zambia examining the impact of maternity waiting homes as a system-based intervention to increase access to quality intrapartum care for women living in remote, rural areas far from a skilled provider. She recently completed the first study of group antenatal care for low- and nonliterate women in sub-Saharan Africa. She holds a Ph.D. in nursing from the University of Arizona and an M.S. in midwifery from the University of Michigan.

Jeanne Miranda, Ph.D., M.S., is a professor in the Department of Psychiatry and Biobehavioral Sciences at University of California, Los Angeles (UCLA). She is a mental health services researcher who has focused her work on providing mental health care to low-income and minority communities. Dr. Miranda's major research contributions have been in evaluating the impact of mental health care for ethnic minority communities. She is currently working with two community partners—TIES for Families and the Center for Adoption Support and Education—to evaluate an intervention her team developed to provide care for families adopting older children from foster care. She is also working to develop appropriate depression interventions for young women in Uganda and evaluating a government microfinance program in Uganda. Dr. Miranda is an investigator in two UCLA centers focused on improving disparities in health care for ethnic minorities. She is a member of the National Academy of Medicine and a recipient of the Emily Mumford Award for Contributions to Social Medicine from Columbia University. She holds a Ph.D. in clinical psychology from the University of Kansas and completed postdoctoral training at the University of California, San Francisco.

Ruth Murphey Parker, M.D., is professor of medicine at the Emory University School of Medicine. She holds secondary appointments in pediatrics and in epidemiology at the university's Rollins School of Public Health and is a senior fellow of the Center for Ethics. Her primary research interests and activities are in health services of underserved populations, particularly health literacy. She recently completed a position as chair of the Nonprescription Drug Advisory Committee for the U.S. Food and Drug Administration (FDA), and has served as an expert in label comprehension for various FDA advisory committees representing issues related to health literacy and patient/consumer understanding of drug information. She is a member of a Patient-Centered Outcomes Research Institute advisory group and serves on an expert panel for the U.S. Pharmacopeia. Dr. Parker was principal investigator in the Robert Wood Johnson Literacy in Health Study and co-authored the Test of Functional Health Literacy in Adults, a measurement tool for quantifying patients' ability to read and understand health information. She chaired the American Medical Association Foundation steering committee for the national program on health literacy and also chaired the American College of Physicians Foundation Patient Literacy Advisory Board. She consults with various federal and state agencies, professional societies, and members of industry regarding their efforts to advance health literacy. She earned her M.D. at the University of North Carolina at Chapel Hill. She holds board certification in both internal medicine and pediatrics and is an appointed associate of the National Research Council.

Deborah E. Powell, M.D., is dean emerita of the medical school and professor in the Department of Laboratory Medicine and Pathology at the University of Minnesota. She joined the university in 2002 and led the University of Minnesota Medical School until 2009. She was also assistant vice president for clinical sciences, associate vice president for new models of education, and McKnight presidential leadership chairman at the University of Minnesota, Twin Cities. Prior to coming to the University of Minnesota, she served as executive dean and vice chancellor for clinical affairs at the University of Kansas School of Medicine for 5 years. Previously, she served as chairman of the Department of Pathology and Laboratory Medicine and as vice chairman and director of diagnostic pathology at the University of Kentucky in Lexington. She is a medical educator and has more than 30 years of experience in academic medicine. Additionally, she has been president of the United States and Canadian Academy of Pathology and president of the American Board of Pathology. She served as chairman of the Council of Deans of the Association of American Medical Colleges and as chair of the Association of American Medical Colleges in 2009–2010. She has served as director of the Accreditation Council for Graduate Medical Education, the Institute for Healthcare Improvement, Fairview Health System, the University of Minnesota Medical Center, the Association of American Medical Colleges, and Hazelden. She is a member of the National Academy of Medicine. Dr. Powell is a board-certified surgical pathologist. She received her medical degree from Tufts University School of Medicine.

Eva K. Pressman, M.D., is Henry A. Thiede Professor and chair of the Department of Obstetrics and Gynecology (OB/GYN) at the University of Rochester. She formerly served as director of maternal fetal medicine (MFM), director of the MFM Fellowship training program, director of reproductive genetics, and director of OB/GYN ultrasound. Before coming to the University of Rochester in 1999, she was an assistant professor at The Johns Hopkins University from 1994 to 1999, where she was also associate director of the OB/GYN Residency Program and director of the Fetal Assessment Center and of the High Risk Obstetrical Clinic. Dr. Pressman is board-certified in OB/GYN and in MFM. Among her current areas of interest are medical complications of pregnancy, including diabetes and psychiatric disorders, and nutrition and metabolism in pregnancy. She received her medical degree at Duke University School of Medicine, where she was elected to Alpha Omega Alpha Honor Society. Dr. Pressman completed her residency training in OB/GYN as well as a fellowship in MFM at Johns Hopkins University.

Alina Salganicoff, Ph.D., is vice president and director of women's health policy at the Kaiser Family Foundation. Widely regarded as an expert on women's health policy, she has written and lectured extensively on health care access and financing for low-income women and their families. Her work focuses on health coverage and access to care for women, with an emphasis on understanding the impact of state and federal policies on underserved women throughout their life span. Dr. Salganicoff was also an associate director of the Kaiser Commission on Medicaid and the Uninsured and worked on the health program staff of The Pew Charitable Trusts. She has served as advisor on women's health issues to numerous federal agencies, including the Department of Veterans Affairs, the Centers for Disease Control and Prevention, the Health Resources and Services Administration, the Agency for Healthcare Research and Quality, and the Department of Health and Human Services' Office of Women's Health. She has also served on many state-level and nonprofit advisory committees. Dr. Salganicoff holds a Ph.D. in health policy from The Johns Hopkins University and a B.S. from The Pennsylvania State University.

Paul G. Shekelle, M.D., Ph.D., M.P.H., is co-director of the Southern California Evidence-based Practice Center at the RAND Corporation. He is a staff physician in internal medicine at the West Los Angeles Veterans Affairs Medical Center and also a professor of medicine at the UCLA School of Medicine. He earned his M.D. from Duke University and his Ph.D. from UCLA.

Susan M. Wolf, J.D., is McKnight Professor of Law, Medicine & Public Policy; Faegre Baker Daniels Professor of Law; and professor of medicine at the University of Minnesota. She is also chair of the university's Consortium on Law and Values in Health, Environment & the Life Sciences. Professor Wolf teaches in the areas of health law, law and science, and bioethics. She is a member of the National Academy of Medicine, a fellow of the American Association for the Advancement of Science, a fellow of The Hastings Center, and a member of the American Law Institute. She has served on a variety of governmental and institutional panels, including the National Science Advisory Board for Biosecurity, the American Society for Reproductive Medicine's Ethics Committee, and the Memorial Sloan-Kettering Cancer Center's Ethics Committee. Professor Wolf currently serves on the National Academies Committee on Science, Engineering, Medicine, and Public Policy. She is a past chair of the Association of American Law Schools Section on Law, Medicine and Health Care and a past board member of the American Society for Bioethics and Humanities. She received her J.D. from Yale Law School.

Appendix B

Acronyms and Glossary

ACRONYMS

AAAASF	American Association for Accreditation of Ambulatory Surgery Facilities
AAAHC	Accreditation Association for Ambulatory Heath Care
AAPA	American Academy of Physician Assistants
ACGME	Accreditation Council for Graduate Medical Education
ACME	Accreditation Commission for Midwifery Education
ACNM	American College of Nurse-Midwives
ACOG	American College of Obstetricians and Gynecologists
AHRQ	Agency for Healthcare Research and Quality
AMCB	American Midwifery Certification Board
ANSIRH	Advancing New Standards in Reproductive Health
APA	American Psychological Association
APAOG	Association of Physician Assistants in Obstetrics & Gynecology
APC	advanced practice clinician
APHA	American Public Health Association
ARC-PA	Accreditation Review Commission on Education for the Physician Assistant
ASA	American Society of Anesthesiologists
ASC	ambulatory surgery center
CAPS	Consortium of Abortion Providers
CDC	U.S. Centers for Disease Control and Prevention
CI	confidence interval

CMS   Centers for Medicare & Medicaid Services
CNM   certified nurse-midwife
CRNA   certified registered nurse anesthetist

D&C   dilation and sharp curettage
D&E   dilation and evacuation

EVA   electric vacuum aspiration

FAERS   FDA Adverse Event Reporting System
FDA   U.S. Food and Drug Administration
FPL   federal poverty level

HWPP   Health Workforce Pilot Project

IOM   Institute of Medicine
IUD   intrauterine device

LMP   last menstrual period

MAC   monitored anesthesia care
MAP   Midwest Access Project
MVA   manual vacuum aspiration

NAF   National Abortion Federation
NCCPA   National Commission on Certification of Physician Assistants
NCI   National Cancer Institute
NONPF   National Organization of Nurse Practitioner Faculties
NP   nurse practitioner

OB/GYN   obstetrician/gynecologist
OSHPD   Office of Statewide Health Planning and Development

PA   physician assistant
PTSD   posttraumatic stress disorder

RCOG   Royal College of Obstetricians and Gynaecologists
RCT   randomized controlled trial
REMS   Risk Evaluation and Mitigation Strategy
RHAP   Reproductive Health Access Project
RHEDI   Reproductive Health Education in Family Medicine

SFP   Society of Family Planning
STFM   Society of Teachers of Family Medicine
STI   sexually transmitted infection

UCSF   University of California, San Francisco

WHO   World Health Organization

GLOSSARY

abortion rate	The annual number of abortions per 1,000 women aged 15–44 or other specific group within a given population.
abortion ratio	The annual number of abortions per 1,000 live births within a given population.
abortion-related death	A death resulting from a direct complication of an abortion (legal or illegal), from an indirect complication caused by a chain of events initiated by an abortion, or from an aggravation of a preexisting condition by the physiological or psychological effects of abortion.
advanced practice clinicians (APCs)	Include physician assistants (PAs), certified nurse-midwives (CNMs), and nurse practitioners (NPs).
aspiration abortion	Also referred to as surgical abortion or suction curettage, this procedure is used up to 14 to 16 weeks' gestation. A hollow curette (tube) is inserted into the uterus. At the other end of the curette, a handheld syringe or an electric device is applied to create suction and empty the uterus.
buccal administration	Administering a drug by placing in between the gums and cheek.
case control study	An observational study that analyzes one group of persons with a certain disease, chronic condition, or type of injury (case patients) and another group of persons without the health problem (control subjects) and compares differences in their exposures, behaviors, and other characteristics to identify and quantify associations, test hypotheses, and identify causes.

case series	Analyses of a series of people with a disease or health condition (there is no comparison group in case series).
certified nurse-midwife (CNM)	An advanced practice registered nurse who has advanced education (master's or doctorate) and training in both midwifery and nursing and is certified by the American Midwifery Certification Board.
cohort studies	Observational studies in which groups of exposed individuals (e.g., women with an abortion in their first pregnancy or women whose early-gestation pregnancy was terminated by aspiration) are compared with groups of unexposed individuals (e.g., women whose first pregnancy was a delivery or women whose early-gestation pregnancy was terminated by medication) and monitored over time to observe an outcome of interest (e.g., future fertility). Cohort studies can be either prospective or retrospective.
comorbidity	A condition that exists at the same time as the primary condition in the same patient (e.g., hypertension is a comorbidity of many conditions, such as diabetes, ischemic heart disease, and end-stage renal disease).
contraception	An agent that prevents ovulation, fertilization of an egg, or implantation of a fertilized egg, thereby preventing a pregnancy from taking place.
deep sedation	A drug-induced depression of consciousness during which patients cannot easily be aroused but respond purposefully following repeated or painful stimulation. The ability to maintain ventilatory function independently may be impaired. Patients may require assistance in maintaining a patent airway, and spontaneous ventilation may be inadequate. Cardiovascular function is usually maintained but may be impaired.
dilation and sharp curettage (D&C)	A surgical procedure in which the cervix is dilated so that the uterine lining can be scraped with a curette to remove products of conception.
dilation and evacuation (D&E)	An abortion procedure that can be performed starting at 14 weeks' gestation. The procedure involves cervical preparation with osmotic dilators and/or medications, followed by suction and/or forceps extraction to empty the uterus. Ultrasound guidance is often used.

ectopic pregnancy	An abnormal pregnancy that occurs when a fertilized egg grows outside of the uterus, most commonly in a fallopian tube. As the pregnancy progresses, it can cause the tube to rupture (burst), which can cause major internal bleeding. This can be life-threatening and needs to be treated with surgery.
effective	Providing services based on scientific knowledge to all who could benefit and refraining from providing services to those not likely to benefit (avoiding underuse and overuse, respectively).
efficient	Avoiding waste, including waste of equipment, supplies, ideas, and energy.
equitable	Providing care that does not vary in quality because of personal characteristics such as gender, ethnicity, geographic location, and socioeconomic status.
general anesthesia	A drug-induced loss of consciousness during which patients are not arousable, even by painful stimulation. The ability to maintain ventilatory function independently is often impaired. Patients often require assistance in maintaining a patent airway, and positive pressure ventilation may be required because of depressed spontaneous ventilation or drug-induced depression of neuromuscular function. Cardiovascular function may be impaired.
hemorrhage	Bleeding in excess of 500 mL and/or excessive bleeding that requires a clinical response, such as transfusion or hospital admission.
incomplete abortion	Occurs when parts of the products of conception are retained in the uterus.
induction abortion	Also referred to as "medical" abortion; involves the use of medications to induce labor and delivery of the fetus. The most effective regimens use a combination of mifepristone and misoprostol.
laminaria	A type of osmotic dilator (see definition below). Laminaria tents are made of dried, compressed Japanese seaweed derived from japonica or digitate plants. Laminaria comes in diameters ranging from 2 to 10 mm, and in the standard 60 mm length as well as an extra-long 85 mm model.

local anesthesia	Elimination or reduction of sensation, especially pain, in one part of the body by topical application or local injection of a drug. In the context of abortion practice, local anesthesia almost always involves a paracervical block.
medication abortion	Also referred to as "medical" abortion; involves the use of medications to induce uterine contractions that expel the products of conception. The regimen, approved by the FDA up to 70 days' gestation, uses 200 mg of mifepristone followed by 800 mcg of misoprostol 24 to 48 hours later.
meta-analysis	A systematic review that uses statistical methods to combine the results of similar studies quantitatively in an attempt to allow inferences to be drawn from the sample of studies and applied to the population of interest.
Mifeprex (mifepristone)	The brand name for mifepristone, a progesterone receptor antagonist that competitively binds to the progesterone receptor, thereby inhibiting the physiological action of progesterone, a hormone needed for a pregnancy to continue. When used together with another medicine called misoprostol (defined below), Mifeprex is used to end a pregnancy.
minimal sedation (anxiolysis)	A drug-induced state during which patients respond normally to verbal commands. Although cognitive function and physical coordination may be impaired, airway reflexes and ventilatory and cardiovascular functions are unaffected.
miscarriage	Also termed spontaneous abortion (see below); the spontaneous loss of a fetus before 20 weeks' gestation. Spontaneous abortion is a naturally occurring event.
misoprostol	A synthetic prostaglandin E1 analogue that is used off-label for a variety of indications in the practice of obstetrics and gynecology, including medication abortion, medical management of miscarriage, induction of labor, cervical ripening before surgical procedures, and the treatment of postpartum hemorrhage. Misoprostol's effects are dose dependent and include cervical softening and dilation, uterine contractions, nausea, vomiting, diarrhea, fever, and chills.

moderate sedation	Also referred to as conscious sedation; a drug-induced depression of consciousness during which patients respond purposefully to verbal commands, either alone or accompanied by light tactile stimulation. No interventions are required to maintain a patent airway, and spontaneous ventilation is adequate. Cardiovascular function is usually maintained.
nurse practitioner (NP)	An advanced practice registered nurse who has advanced education (typically a master's degree) and extensive clinical training in both the NP role (e.g., acute or primary care) and one or more population practice areas (e.g., family, women's health) and specialty practice areas (e.g., high-risk perinatal, infertility, abortion care). NPs diagnose and manage patient care for many acute and chronic illnesses, and they also provide preventive care.
osmotic dilator	A device that absorbs moisture from the tissues surrounding the cervix and swells, slowly opening the cervix. There are two common types of osmotic dilators: laminaria, a small tube made of dried seaweed (see above), and synthetic dilators, tubes with varying rigidity and size made of polymer.
patient-centered	Defined as "providing care that is respectful of and responsive to individual patient preferences, needs, and values and ensuring that patient values guide all clinical decisions."
physician assistant (PA)	An individual certified to practice medicine with physician supervision (indirect). They provide health care services that range from primary care to very specialized surgical services.
safety	Avoiding injuries to patients from the care that is intended to help them.
spontaneous abortion	The spontaneous loss of a fetus before 20 weeks' gestation. Spontaneous abortion is a naturally occurring event.
surgical abortion	A term used to describe aspiration and dilation and evacuation (D&E) procedures. This report uses the specific procedure terms to avoid confusion as to what procedure is being described.

systematic review	A scientific investigation that focuses on a specific question and that uses explicit, planned scientific methods to identify, select, assess, and summarize the findings of similar but separate studies. It may or may not include a quantitative synthesis of the results from separate studies (meta-analysis, defined above).
timely	Reducing waits and sometimes harmful delays for both those who receive and those who give care.
unsafe abortion	A procedure for terminating an unintended pregnancy carried out either by persons lacking the necessary skills or in an environment that does not conform to minimal medical standards, or both.
uterine perforation	A rupture in the uterus caused by traumatic or pathologic processes.

Appendix C

Public Meeting Agenda

Workshop on Facility Standards and the Safety of Outpatient Procedures

March 24, 2017
Keck Center of the National Academies
Room 100
500 Fifth Street NW
Washington, DC

Workshop Objective: To learn about accreditation and other facility standards that relate to delivering abortion services.

8:30 a.m.   **Welcome and Introductory Remarks**

Ned Calonge, M.D., M.P.H., Committee Co-Chair

8:40 a.m.   **Meeting Accreditation and State Licensing Requirements: The Experiences of Provider Organizations**

Juliet Rogers, Ph.D., M.P.H., Assistant Professor, Health Management and Policy, University of Michigan

Q&A/Discussion

9:20 a.m.   **Differences in Facility Standards: Abortions and Other Outpatient Procedures**

Bonnie Scott Jones, J.D., Senior Policy Advisor, Advancing New Standards in Reproductive Health (ANSIRH), University of California, San Francisco

Q&A/Discussion

10:00 a.m. **Research on the Relationship of Facility-Related Factors and Patient Outcomes for Non-Hospital-Based Outpatient Procedures**

Sarah Roberts, Dr.P.H., Associate Professor, Advancing New Standards in Reproductive Health (ANSIRH), Department of Obstetrics, Gynecology, and Reproductive Sciences, University of California, San Francisco

Q&A/Discussion

10:45 a.m. **Break**

11:00 a.m. **Public Comments (3–5 minutes each)**

Q&A/Discussion

12:00 p.m. **Closing Remarks**

Helene Gayle, M.D., M.P.H., Committee Co-Chair

12:10 p.m. **Adjourn**

Appendix D

Literature Search Strategy

Professional research librarians conducted literature searches for this study based on the statement of task and reference interviews with program staff and the committee to identify relevant research. The databases that were searched included Medline, Embase, PubMed, Scopus, PsycINFO, CINAHL, Web of Science, and Cochrane Database of Systematic Reviews. Titles and abstracts identified in the literature searches were organized into EndNote libraries.

Table D-1 broadly details the scope of each search. The search syntax for each literature search is detailed in the sections below.

TABLE D-1 Literature Searches

Topic	Date	Literature	Date Range	Databases	No. of Citations Yielded
Mental Health Outcomes	2/8/2017	Systematic Reviews, Meta-Analysis	2000–Present	Medline, Embase, Cochrane, PubMed, PsycINFO	142
Short-Term Health Effects	2/8/2017	Systematic Reviews, Meta-Analysis	2000–Present	Medline, Embase, Cochrane, PubMed	248
Mental Health Outcomes	3/2/2017	Primary Literature, Editorials	2000–Present	Medline, Embase, PubMed, PsycINFO	460
Short-Term Health Effects	3/2/2017	Primary Literature, Editorials	2012–Present	Medline, Embase, PubMed,	617
Disparities	3/3/2017	Systematic Reviews, Meta-Analysis, Primary Literature, Editorials	2000–Present	Medline, Embase, PubMed, Scopus	1,381
Long-Term Health Effects	3/30/2017	Systematic Reviews, Meta-Analysis, Primary Literature, Editorials	1970–Present	Medline, Embase, PubMed	2,072
Delays	4/19/2017	Systematic Reviews, Meta-Analysis, Primary Literature, Editorials	2005–Present	Medline, Embase, PubMed Web of Science	1,259
Cancer	6/19/2017	Systematic Reviews, Meta-Analysis, Primary Literature, Editorials	2007–Present	Medline, Embase, Cochrane, PubMed	1,835
Training	2/20/2017	Systematic Reviews, Meta-Analysis, Primary Literature, Editorials	2000–Present	PubMed, CINAHL, Cochrane	1,378

MENTAL HEALTH OUTCOMES

Systematic Reviews

Search Strategy: Mental Health Outcomes
Date: 2000–Present
Countries: United States and International
Population: Human
Document Types: Systematic Reviews, Meta-Analysis
Databases Searched: Medline, Embase, Cochrane, PubMed, and PsycINFO

Search No.	Search Syntax
Medline (Ovid)	
1	Abortion Applicants/ or Abortion, Induced/
2	Mental Disorders/ or Mental Health/
3	Depression/
4	Anxiety/
5	(mental health or distress or relief or depression or counseling).ti,ab.
6	or/2–5
7	Animals/
8	(animal or animals or mice or mouse or rat or rats).ti,ab.
9	or/7–8
10	Abortion, Spontaneous/
11	spontaneous abortion.ti,ab.
12	or/10–11
13	Adolescent/
14	under 18.ti,ab.
15	(adolescent or adolescents or teenager or teen).ti,ab.
16	or/13–15
17	1 and 6
18	17 not 9
19	18 not 12
20	19
21	limit 20 to yr="2000–Current"
22	limit 21 to ("review" or systematic reviews)
23	22 and 16
24	geographic variation.ti,ab.
25	Regional Medical Programs/
26	Residence Characteristics/
27	Health Services Accessibility/
28	United States/
29	appalachian region/ or great lakes region/ or mid-atlantic region/ or midwestern united states/ or new england/ or northwestern united states/ or pacific states/ or southeastern united states/ or southwestern united states/
30	or/24–29
31	22 and 30
32	Socioeconomic Factors/
33	Poverty/ or Social Class/
34	socioeconomic status.ti,ab.
35	or/32–34
36	22 and 35

37	Continental Population Groups/
38	Ethnic Groups/
39	African Americans/
40	asian americans/ or hispanic americans/
41	(race or ethnicity).ti,ab.
42	or/37–41
43	22 and 42
44	22

Embase (Ovid)

1	Abortion Applicants/ or Abortion, Induced/
2	Mental Disorders/ or Mental Health/
3	Depression/
4	Anxiety/
5	(mental health or distress or relief or depression or counseling).ti,ab.
6	or/2–5
7	Animals/
8	(animal or animals or mice or mouse or rat or rats).ti,ab.
9	or/7–8
10	Abortion, Spontaneous/
11	spontaneous abortion.ti,ab.
12	or/10–11
13	Adolescent/
14	under 18.ti,ab.
15	(adolescent or adolescents or teenager or teen).ti,ab.
16	or/13–15
17	1 and 6
18	17 not 9
19	18 not 12
20	19
21	limit 20 to yr="2000–Current"
22	limit 21 to ("review")
23	22 and 16
24	geographic variation.ti,ab.
25	Regional Medical Programs/
26	Residence Characteristics/
27	Health Services Accessibility/
28	United States/
29	appalachian region/ or great lakes region/ or mid-atlantic region/ or midwestern united states/ or new england/ or northwestern united states/ or pacific states/ or southeastern united states/ or southwestern united states/
30	or/24–29
31	22 and 30
32	Socioeconomic Factors/
33	Poverty/ or Social Class/
34	socioeconomic status.ti,ab.
35	or/32–34
36	22 and 35
37	Continental Population Groups/
38	Ethnic Groups/
39	African Americans/
40	asian americans/ or hispanic americans/

41	(race or ethnicity).ti,ab.
42	or/37–41
43	22 and 42
44	22

Cochrane Database of Systematic Reviews (Ovid)

1	abortion.ti,ab.
2	mental health.ti,ab.
3	(mental disorder or distress or grief or depression or counseling or anxiety). ti,ab.
4	or/2–3
5	1 and 4

PubMed:
Note: The following search was run to capture e-pub ahead of print, under indexed and recent articles not yet indexed in Medline.
("Abortion, Induced"[Mesh] OR abortion [Title/Abstract])
Filters: Review, Systematic Reviews, Publication date from 206/01/01 to 2017/12/31, Humans

PsycINFO (ProQuest):
SU.EXACT("Induced Abortion") AND (SU.EXACT("Anxiety") OR SU.EXACT("Posttraumatic Stress Disorder") OR SU.EXACT("Depression (Emotion)") OR SU.EXACT("Post-Traumatic Stress") OR SU.EXACT("Major Depression") OR SU.EXACT("Anxiety Disorders") OR SU.EXACT("Stress") OR SU.EXACT("Psychological Stress") OR SU.EXACT("Mental Disorders") OR SU.EXACT("Grief") OR anxiety OR stress OR depression OR grief OR "mental disorder" OR "mental health")
Limits:
Date: After January 1, 2000
Document type: Journal, Journal Article, Peer Reviewed Journal, Peer-reviewed Journal
Methodology: Literature Review, Longitudinal Study, Meta-Analysis, Meta Synthesis, Systematic Review
Population: Human

Primary Literature

Search Strategy: Mental Health Outcomes
Date: 2000–Present
Countries: United States and International
Population: Human
Document Types: Primary Literature, Editorials
Databases Searched: Medline, Embase, PubMed, and PsycINFO

Search No.	Search Syntax
Embase (Ovid)	
1	induced abortion/ or (induced adj abortion).ti,kw.
2	mental disease/ or acute stress/ or physical stress/ or posttraumatic stress disorder/ or stress/ or emotional stress/ or acute stress disorder/ or physiological stress/

3	mental health/
4	depression/
5	anxiety/
6	grief/
7	(mental health or distress or depression or anxiety or grief or stress or ptsd or post traumatic stress disorder).kw.
8	or/2–7
9	1 and 8
10	spontaneous abortion/
11	(spontaneous adj abortion).kw.
12	or/10–11
13	9 not 12
14	animal/
15	(animal or animals or mice or mouse or rat or rats).kw.
16	or/14–15
17	13 not 16
18	17
19	limit 18 to yr="2000–Current"
20	limit 19 to (editorial or letter or note)
21	limit 19 to (article or conference abstract or conference paper or conference proceeding or "conference review" or journal or report or short survey or trade journal)
22	21 not 20

Medline (Ovid)

1	Abortion, Induced/ or (induced adj abortion).kw,ti.
2	Mental Disorders/ or Mental Health/
3	Depression/
4	Anxiety/ or Stress Disorders, Post-Traumatic/ or Stress Disorders, Traumatic/ or Stress Disorders, Traumatic, Acute/ or Stress, Psychological/ or Stress, Physiological/ or Grief/
5	(mental health or distress or depression or anxiety or grief or stress or ptsd or post traumatic stress disorder).kw.
6	or/2–5
7	Animals/
8	(animal or animals or mice or mouse or rat or rats).kw.
9	or/7–8
10	Abortion, Spontaneous/
11	(spontaneous adj abortion).kw.
12	or/10–11
13	1 and 6
14	13 not 9
15	14 not 12
16	15
17	limit 16 to yr="2000–Current"
18	limit 17 to (comment or editorial or guideline or letter or news)
19	limit 17 to (case reports or classical article or clinical study or clinical trial, all or clinical trial, phase i or clinical trial, phase ii or clinical trial, phase iii or clinical trial, phase iv or clinical trial or comparative study or controlled clinical trial or evaluation studies or historical article or journal article or meta analysis or multicenter study or observational study or pragmatic

clinical trial or randomized controlled trial or technical report or twin study or validation studies)

20   19 not 18

PsycINFO (ProQuest):
(SU.EXACT("Induced Abortion")) AND (SU.EXACT("Anxiety") OR SU.EXACT("Posttraumatic Stress Disorder") OR SU.EXACT("Depression (Emotion)") OR SU.EXACT("Post-Traumatic Stress") OR SU.EXACT("Major Depression") OR SU.EXACT("Anxiety Disorders") OR SU.EXACT("Stress") OR SU.EXACT("Psychological Stress") OR SU.EXACT("Mental Disorders") OR SU.EXACT("Grief"))
Limits:
Date: After January 1, 2000
Record type: Comment/Reply OR Editorial OR Letter
Record type: Journal OR Peer Reviewed Journal OR Journal Article OR Peer-reviewed Journal

PubMed:
Note: The following search was run to capture e-pub ahead of print, under indexed and recent articles not yet in Medline.
("Abortion, Induced"[Mesh] OR abortion[tw]) AND (mental health[tw] OR "Mental Health"[Mesh])

SHORT-TERM HEALTH EFFECTS

Systematic Reviews

Search Strategy: Short-Term Health Effects
Date: 2000–Present
Countries: United States and International
Population: Human
Document Types: Systematic Reviews, Meta-Analysis
Databases Searched: Medline, Embase, Cochrane, and PubMed

Search No.	Search Syntax
Medline (Ovid)	
1	Abortion, Induced/
2	abortion.ti,ab.
3	1 or 2
4	Mortality/
5	Hospitalization/
6	Emergency Service, Hospital/
7	Blood Transfusion/ or Blood Component Transfusion/
8	Infection/
9	Antibiotic Prophylaxis/
10	Postoperative Complications/
11	(mortality or hospitalization or emergency room or transfusion or infection or prophylactic antibiotics or surgery or abortion complications or short term effects).ti,ab.

12	or/4–11
13	3 and 12
14	Animals/
15	Mice/
16	Rats/
17	(animal or animals or mice or mouse or rat or rats).ti,ab.
18	or/14–17
19	13 not 18
20	limit 19 to ("review" or systematic reviews)
21	Adolescent/
22	under 18.ti,ab.
23	(adolescent or adolescents or teenager or teen).ti,ab.
24	or/21–23
25	20 and 24
26	Abortion, Spontaneous/
27	spontaneous abortion.ti,ab.
28	or/26-27
29	25 not 28
30	29
31	limit 29 to yr="2000–Current"
32	geographic variation.ti,ab.
33	Regional Medical Programs/
34	Residence Characteristics/
35	Health Services Accessibility/
36	United States/
37	appalachian region/ or great lakes region/ or mid-atlantic region/ or midwestern united states/ or new england/ or northwestern united states/ or pacific states/ or southeastern united states/ or southwestern united states/
38	or/32–37
39	20 and 38
40	39 not 28
41	40
42	limit 41 to yr="2000–Current"
43	Socioeconomic Factors/
44	Poverty/ or Social Class/
45	socioeconomic status.ti,ab.
46	or/43–45
47	20 and 46
48	47 not 28
49	48
50	limit 49 to yr="2000–Current"
51	Continental Population Groups/
52	Ethnic Groups/
53	African Americans/
54	asian americans/ or hispanic americans/
55	(race or ethnicity).ti,ab.
56	or/51–55
57	20 and 56
58	57 not 28
59	58
60	limit 59 to yr="2000–Current"
61	1 and 12

62	61
63	limit 62 to yr="2000–Current"
64	63 not 18
65	limit 64 to ("review" or systematic reviews)

Embase (Ovid)

1	Abortion, Induced/
2	abortion.ti,ab.
3	1 or 2
4	Mortality/
5	Hospitalization/
6	Emergency Service, Hospital/
7	Blood Transfusion/ or Blood Component Transfusion/
8	Infection/
9	Antibiotic Prophylaxis/
10	Postoperative Complications/
11	(mortality or hospitalization or emergency room or transfusion or infection or prophylactic antibiotics or surgery or abortion complications or short term effects).ti,ab.
12	or/4–11
13	3 and 12
14	Animals/
15	Mice/
16	Rats/
17	(animal or animals or mice or mouse or rat or rats).ti,ab.
18	or/14–17
19	13 not 18
20	limit 19 to ("review")
21	Adolescent/
22	under 18.ti,ab.
23	(adolescent or adolescents or teenager or teen).ti,ab.
24	or/21–23
25	20 and 24
26	Abortion, Spontaneous/
27	spontaneous abortion.ti,ab.
28	or/26–27
29	25 not 28
30	29
31	limit 29 to yr="2000–Current"
32	geographic variation.ti,ab.
33	Regional Medical Programs/
34	Residence Characteristics/
35	Health Services Accessibility/
36	United States/
37	appalachian region/ or great lakes region/ or mid-atlantic region/ or midwestern united states/ or new england/ or northwestern united states/ or pacific states/ or southeastern united states/ or southwestern united states/
38	or/32–37
39	20 and 38
40	39 not 28
41	40
42	limit 41 to yr="2000–Current"

43	Socioeconomic Factors/
44	Poverty/ or Social Class/
45	socioeconomic status.ti,ab.
46	or/43–45
47	20 and 46
48	47 not 28
49	48
50	limit 49 to yr="2000–Current"
51	Continental Population Groups/
52	Ethnic Groups/
53	African Americans/
54	asian americans/ or hispanic americans/
55	(race or ethnicity).ti,ab.
56	or/51–55
57	20 and 56
58	57 not 28
59	58
60	limit 59 to yr="2000–Current"
61	1 and 12
62	61
63	limit 62 to yr="2000–Current"
64	63 not 18
65	limit 64 to ("review")

Cochrane Database of Systematic Reviews (Ovid)

1	abortion.ti,ab.
2	short term effects.ti,ab.
3	(mortality or hospitalization or emergency room or transfusion or infection or prophylactic antibiotics or surgery or complications).ti,ab.
4	or/2–3
5	1 and 4

PubMed:

Note: The following search was run to capture e-pub ahead of print, under indexed and recent articles not yet in Medline.

("Abortion, Induced"[Mesh] OR abortion [Title/Abstract])

Filters: Review, Systematic Reviews, Publication date from 206/01/01 to 2017/12/31, Humans

Primary Literature

Search Strategy: Short-Term Effects
Date: 2012–Present
Countries: United States and International
Population: Human
Document Types: Primary Literature, Editorials
Databases Searched: Medline, Embase, and PubMed

Search No.	Search Syntax

Medline (Ovid)

1	Abortion, Induced/ or (induced adj abortion).kw,ti. or Abortion, Induced/ co [Complications]
2	Mortality/
3	Hospitalization/
4	Emergency Service, Hospital/
5	Blood Transfusion/ or Blood Component Transfusion/
6	Infection/
7	Antibiotic Prophylaxis/
8	Postoperative Complications/ or Pain/
9	(mortality or hospitalization or emergency room or transfusion or infection or antibiotics or surgery or pain or complications).kw.
10	or/2–9
11	1 and 10
12	Abortion, Spontaneous/ or (spontaneous adj abortion).kw.
13	11 not 12
14	Animals/ or (animal or animals or mice or mouse or rat or rats).kw.
15	13 not 14
16	15
17	limit 16 to yr="2012–Current"
18	limit 17 to (comment or editorial or guideline or letter or news)
19	limit 17 to (case reports or classical article or clinical study or clinical trial, all or clinical trial, phase i or clinical trial, phase ii or clinical trial, phase iii or clinical trial, phase iv or clinical trial or comparative study or controlled clinical trial or evaluation studies or historical article or journal article or meta analysis or multicenter study or observational study or pragmatic clinical trial or randomized controlled trial or technical report or twin study or validation studies)
20	19 not 18

Embase (Ovid)

1	induced abortion/ or (induced adj abortion).ti,kw.
2	mortality/
3	hospitalization/
4	emergency ward/
5	emergency health service/
6	blood transfusion/
7	intrauterine infection/ or infection/
8	pain/
9	pain/co [Complication]
10	antibiotic agent/
11	postoperative complication/
12	(mortality or hospitalization or emergency room or transfusion or infection or antibiotics or surgery or pain or complications).kw.
13	or/2–12
14	1 and 13
15	spontaneous abortion/
16	(spontaneous adj abortion).kw.
17	or/15–16
18	14 not 17

19	animal/
20	(animal or animals or mice or mouse or rat or rats).kw.
21	or/19–20
22	18 not 21
23	22
24	limit 23 to yr="2012–Current"
25	limit 24 to (editorial or letter or note)
26	limit 24 to (article or conference abstract or conference paper or conference proceeding or "conference review" or journal or report or short survey or trade journal)
27	26 not 25

PubMed:
("Abortion, Induced/adverse effects"[Mesh] OR "Abortion, Induced/complications"[Mesh])
Limit: 2012–Current
("Abortion, Induced"[Mesh] OR abortion[Title/Textword]) AND (complications [Title/Textword] OR "Postoperative Complications"[Mesh])
Limit: 2015–Current

DISPARITIES

Systematic Reviews and Primary Literature

Search Strategy: Disparities
Date: 2000–Present
Countries: United States and International
Population: Human
Document Types: Primary Literature, Editorials, Systematic Reviews, Meta-Analysis
Databases Searched: Medline, Embase, PubMed, and Scopus

Search No.	Search Syntax
Medline (Ovid)	
1	Abortion, Induced/ or (induced adj abortion).kw,ti.
2	Abortion, Spontaneous/
3	(spontaneous adj abortion).kw.
4	or/2–3
5	1 not 4
6	Health Services Accessibility/
7	Health Status Disparities/ or Socioeconomic Factors/ or Healthcare Disparities/
8	disparit*.kw,ti.
9	(geographic adj variation).ti,kw.
10	Poverty Areas/ or Poverty/
11	poverty.ti,kw.
12	Continental Population Groups/
13	Ethnic Groups/
14	(race or ethnicity).kw,ti.
15	Gender Identity/
16	gender.kw,ti.

17	disability.ti,kw.
18	Rural Health/ or Rural Health Services/
19	Urban Health/ or Urban Health Services/
20	(urban or rural).ti,kw.
21	or/6–20
22	5 and 21
23	22
24	limit 23 to yr="2000–Current"
25	United States/
26	United States.ti,kw.
27	or/25–26
28	24 and 27
29	limit 28 to (comment or editorial or guideline or letter or news)
30	28 not 29
31	Texas/
32	texas.kw,ti.
33	or/31–32
34	24 and 33
35	24 not (28 or 34)
36	limit 35 to (comment or editorial or guideline or letter or news)
37	35 not 36

Embase (Ovid)

1	induced abortion/ or (induced adj abortion).ti,kw.
2	spontaneous abortion/
3	(spontaneous adj abortion).ti,kw.
4	or/2–3
5	1 not 4
6	health disparity/
7	health care disparity/
8	social status/
9	disparit*.kw,ti.
10	(geographic adj variation).ti,kw.
11	poverty/
12	poverty.ti,kw.
13	race difference/ or race/
14	ethnic group/ or ethnicity/ or "ethnic or racial aspects"/
15	(race or ethnicity).kw,ti.
16	gender identity/
17	gender.kw,ti.
18	disability/
19	disability.ti,kw.
20	rural area/ or urban area/ or urban rural difference/ or urban population/ or rural population/
21	(urban or rural).ti,kw.
22	or/6–21
23	5 and 22
24	23
25	limit 24 to yr="2000–Current"
26	United States/
27	united states.ti,kw.
28	or/26–27

29	25 and 28
30	limit 29 to (editorial or letter or note)
31	29 not 30
32	limit 25 to (editorial or letter or note)
33	32 not 30
34	25 not 31

Scopus:
Title, Abstract, Keyword searches from 2000–Present:
"abortion disparities"
"induced abortion" AND ("geographic variation" OR "urban" OR "rural")
"induced abortion" AND (inequality OR inequalities)
"induced abortion" AND delay
"induced abortion" AND "socioeconomic status"
"abortion" AND "health disparities"
PubMed:
("Abortion, Induced"[Mesh] OR "induced abortion"[tw]) AND ("Health Status Disparities"[Mesh] AND "Healthcare Disparities"[Mesh] OR "disparity"[tw] OR "disparities"[tw])

LONG-TERM HEALTH EFFECTS

Systematic Reviews and Primary Literature

Search Strategy: Long-Term Health Effects
Date: 1970–Present
Countries: United States and International
Population: Human
Document Types: Primary Literature, Editorials, Systematic Reviews, Meta-Analysis
Databases Searched: Medline, Embase, and PubMed

Search No.	Search Syntax
Embase and Medline (Ovid)	
1	Birth Weight/
2	Breast Neoplasms/
3	Fetal Death/
4	Fetal Membranes, Premature Rupture/
5	Infant, Low Birth Weight/
6	Infant, Newborn/co [Complications]
7	Infant, Premature/
8	Infant, Small for Gestational Age/
9	Infant, Very Low Birth Weight/
10	Infertility, Female/co [Complications]
11	Obstetric Labor Complications/et [Etiology]
12	Obstetric Labor, Premature/
13	Placenta Previa/et [Etiology]
14	[Placenta/ab [Abnormalities]]
15	Pre-Eclampsia/co [Complications]
16	Pregnancy Complications/
17	Pregnancy Outcome/

18	Pregnancy, Ectopic/
19	Pregnancy, High-Risk/
20	Pregnancy, Prolonged/
21	Premature Birth/
22	Uterine Cervical Incompetence/co [Complications]
23	Uterine Hemorrhage/co [Complications]
24	*Abortion, Induced/
25	(induced adj abortion).ti,kw.
26	24 or 25
27	Animals/
28	(animal or animals or mice or mouse or rat or rats).ti,kw.
29	or/27–28
30	(infertility or "cancer risk" or "intrauterine growth" or "future pregnancy" or "fetal growth" or "preterm birth" or premature or "ectopic pregnancy") ti,kw.
31	or/1–23
32	30 or 31
33	26 and 32
34	33 not 29
35	34
36	limit 35 to yr="1970–Current"
37	limit 36 to (meta analysis or "systematic review")
38	limit 36 to (editorial or note)
39	36 not (37 or 38)

PubMed:
(("Abortion, Induced/adverse effects"[Majr] OR abortion [title]) NOT spontaneous [title]) AND (Birth Weight [Mesh] OR Breast Neoplasms [Mesh] OR Fetal Death [Mesh] OR Fetal Membranes, Premature Rupture [Mesh] OR Infant, Low Birth Weight [Mesh] OR Infant, Newborn [Mesh] OR Infant, Premature [Mesh] OR Infant, Small for Gestational Age [Mesh] OR Infant, Very Low Birth Weight [Mesh] OR Infertility, Female/complications [Mesh] OR Obstetric Labor Complications/ etiology*[Mesh] OR Obstetric Labor, Premature [Mesh] OR Placenta Previa/etiology [Mesh] OR Placenta/abnormalities [Mesh] OR Pre-Eclampsia/complications [Mesh] OR Pregnancy Complications [Mesh] OR Pregnancy Outcome[Mesh] OR Pregnancy, Ectopic[Mesh] OR Pregnancy, High-Risk[Mesh] OR Pregnancy, Prolonged[Mesh] OR Premature Birth[Mesh] OR Uterine Cervical Incompetence/complications[Mesh] OR Uterine Hemorrhage/etiology[Mesh])
Limit: 1970–Present
Limit: Humans

DELAYS

Systematic Reviews and Primary Literature

Search Strategy: Delays
Date: 2005–Present
Countries: United States and International
Population: Human
Document Types: Primary Literature, Editorials, Systematic Reviews, Meta-Analysis
Databases Searched: Medline, Embase, and PubMed

Search No.	Search Syntax
Medline (Ovid)	
1	Abortion, Induced/ or (induced adj abortion).ab,ti.
2	Animals/
3	(animal or animals or mice or mouse or rat or rats).ti,ab.
4	or/2–3
5	Abortion, Spontaneous/
6	(spontaneous adj abortion).ti,ab.
7	or/5–6
8	1 not 4
9	8 not 7
10	Health Services Accessibility/
11	Health Facility Closure/
12	Time Factors/
13	Supreme Court Decisions/
14	Texas/
15	Waiting Lists/
16	"waiting periods".ti,ab.
17	"financial issues".ti,ab.
18	"nearest facility".ti,ab.
19	"clinic closure".ti,ab.
20	(distance or restriction or delay or barrier).ti,ab.
21	or/10–20
22	9 and 21
23	22
24	limit 23 to yr="2005–Current"
25	limit 24 to (meta analysis or "review" or systematic reviews)
26	limit 24 to (comment or editorial or letter)
27	24 not (25 or 26)

Search No.	Search Syntax
Embase (Ovid)	
1	*Abortion, Induced/
2	(induced adj abortion).ti,ab.
3	1 or 2
4	Animals/
5	(animal or animals or mice or mouse or rat or rats).ti,ab.
6	or/4–5
7	spontaneous abortion/
8	(spontaneous adj abortion).ti,ab.
9	or/7–8
10	3 not 6
11	10 not 9
12	health care delivery/
13	health care facility/
14	time factor/
15	Texas/
16	hospital admission/
17	"waiting list".ti,ab.
18	"waiting period".ti,ab.
19	"financial issues".ti,ab.

20	"nearest facility".ti,ab.
21	"clinic closure".ti,ab.
22	"supreme court decision".ti,ab.
23	(distance or restriction or delay or barrier).ti,ab.
24	or/12–23
25	11 and 24
26	25
27	limit 26 to yr="2005–Current"
28	limit 27 to (meta analysis or "systematic review")
29	limit 27 to (editorial or letter or note)
30	27 not (28 or 29)

PubMed:
("Abortion, Induced"[Mesh] OR "abortion"[tw]) AND ("waiting period" OR "waiting list" OR "financial issue" OR "nearest facility" OR "clinic closure" OR "Supreme Court decision" OR distance* OR restriction* OR delay* or barrier*) NOT (spontaneous)
Limit: 2005–Current

Database Searched and Time Period Covered:
PubMed: 1/1/2000–4/5/2017

Language:
English

Search Strategy:
"Abortion, Induced"[Mesh] OR abortion, legal[mh] OR abortion*[tiab] OR abortion*[ot]
AND
time factors[mh] OR wait OR waiting OR ban OR bans OR banned OR banning OR barrier* OR deterrent* OR deter OR deterring OR deters OR deterred OR requirement* OR restrict* OR consent* OR difficulty OR difficulties OR limitation* OR confidential* OR privacy OR delay* OR travel* OR distance*
AND
experienc* OR perception* OR perceiv* OR implication* OR impact* OR perspective* OR influen* OR knowledge OR consequence*
AND
AL[Affiliation] OR AK[Affiliation] OR AZ[Affiliation] OR AR[Affiliation] OR CA[Affiliation] OR CO[Affiliation] OR CT[Affiliation] OR DE[Affiliation] OR FL[Affiliation] OR GA[Affiliation] OR HI[Affiliation] OR ID[Affiliation] OR IL[Affiliation] OR IN[Affiliation] OR IA[Affiliation] OR KS[Affiliation] OR KY[Affiliation] OR LA[Affiliation] OR ME[Affiliation] OR MD[Affiliation] OR MA[Affiliation] OR MI[Affiliation] OR MN[Affiliation] OR MS[Affiliation] OR MO[Affiliation] OR MT[Affiliation] OR NE[Affiliation] OR NV[Affiliation] OR NH[Affiliation] OR NJ[Affiliation] OR NM[Affiliation] OR NY[Affiliation] OR NC[Affiliation] OR ND[Affiliation] OR OH[Affiliation] OR OK[Affiliation] OR OR[Affiliation] OR PA[Affiliation] OR RI[Affiliation] OR SC[Affiliation] OR SD[Affiliation] OR TN[Affiliation] OR TX[Affiliation] OR UT[Affiliation] OR VT[Affiliation] OR VA[Affiliation] OR WA[Affiliation] OR WV[Affiliation] OR WI[Affiliation] OR WY[Affiliation] OR USA[AFFILIATION] OR (Alabama[Affiliation] OR Alaska[Affiliation] OR Arizona[Affiliation] OR Arkansas[Affiliation] OR California[Affiliation] OR Colorado[Affiliation] OR Connecticut[Affiliation]

OR Delaware[Affiliation] OR Florida[Affiliation] OR Georgia[Affiliation]
OR Hawaii[Affiliation] OR Idaho[Affiliation] OR Illinois[Affiliation]
OR Indiana[Affiliation] OR Iowa[Affiliation] OR Kansas[Affiliation] OR
Kentucky[Affiliation] OR Louisiana[Affiliation] OR Maine[Affiliation] OR
Maryland[Affiliation] OR Massachusetts[Affiliation] OR Michigan[Affiliation] OR
Minnesota[Affiliation] OR Mississippi[Affiliation] OR Missouri[Affiliation] OR
Montana[Affiliation] OR Nebraska[Affiliation] OR Nevada[Affiliation] OR New
Hampshire[Affiliation] OR New Jersey[Affiliation] OR New Mexico[Affiliation] OR
New York[Affiliation] OR North Carolina[Affiliation] OR North Dakota[Affiliation]
OR Ohio[Affiliation] OR Oklahoma[Affiliation] OR Oregon[Affiliation] OR
Pennsylvania[Affiliation] OR Rhode Island[Affiliation] OR South Carolina[Affiliation]
OR South Dakota[Affiliation] OR Tennessee[Affiliation] OR Texas[Affiliation]
OR Utah[Affiliation] OR Vermont[Affiliation] OR Virginia[Affiliation] OR
Washington[Affiliation] OR West Virginia[Affiliation] OR Wisconsin[Affiliation] OR
Wyoming[Affiliation] OR united states[Affiliation]

Database Searched and Time Period Covered:
Web of Science: 1/1/2000–4/5/2017

Language:
English

Search Strategy: (Note: "TS" = Topic Search)
ts= (abortion*)
AND
ts=(time OR times OR wait OR waiting OR ban OR bans OR banned OR banning
OR barrier* OR deterrent* OR deter OR deterring OR deters OR deterred OR
requirement* OR restrict* OR consent* OR difficulty OR difficulties OR limitation*
OR confidential* OR privacy OR delay* OR travel* OR distance*)
AND
ts=(experienc* OR perception* OR perceiv* OR implication* OR impact* OR
perspective* OR influen* OR knowledge OR consequence*)
AND
COUNTRIES/TERRITORIES: (USA)
NOT
RESEARCH AREAS: (DEVELOPMENTAL BIOLOGY OR MICROBIOLOGY
OR EVOLUTIONARY BIOLOGY OR CELL BIOLOGY OR MARINE
FRESHWATER BIOLOGY OR FORESTRY OR FOOD SCIENCE TECHNOLOGY
OR ENTOMOLOGY OR ENGINEERING OR ENVIRONMENTAL SCIENCES
ECOLOGY OR ACOUSTICS OR VETERINARY SCIENCES OR WATER
RESOURCES OR TROPICAL MEDICINE OR TRANSPLANTATION OR PLANT
SCIENCES OR BIODIVERSITY CONSERVATION OR SPORT SCIENCES
OR RHEUMATOLOGY OR ZOOLOGY OR PHYSIOLOGY OR MEDICAL
LABORATORY TECHNOLOGY OR AGRICULTURE OR DERMATOLOGY OR
PARASITOLOGY OR ALLERGY)
NOT
WEB OF SCIENCE CATEGORIES: (ENDOCRINOLOGY METABOLISM OR
GASTROENTEROLOGY HEPATOLOGY OR VIROLOGY OR PERIPHERAL
VASCULAR DISEASE OR ONCOLOGY OR CARDIAC CARDIOVASCULAR
SYSTEMS OR BIOCHEMICAL RESEARCH METHODS OR ANESTHESIOLOGY
OR UROLOGY NEPHROLOGY OR HEMATOLOGY OR RADIOLOGY NUCLEAR
MEDICINE MEDICAL IMAGING OR IMMUNOLOGY OR BIOTECHNOLOGY

APPLIED MICROBIOLOGY OR GENETICS HEREDITY OR COMPUTER SCIENCE
SOFTWARE ENGINEERING OR COMPUTER SCIENCE INTERDISCIPLINARY
APPLICATIONS OR COMPUTER SCIENCE INFORMATION SYSTEMS OR
BIOCHEMISTRY MOLECULAR BIOLOGY)

Database Searched and Time Period Covered:
Embase: 1/1/2000–5/10/2017

Language:
English

Search Strategy:
"induced abortion"/exp OR abortion*:ab OR abortion*:ti
AND
ban:ti OR bans:ab OR bans:ti OR banned:ab OR banned:ti OR banning:ab OR
banning:ti OR barrier*:ab OR barrier*:ti OR deter*:ab OR deter*:ti OR requir*:ab
OR requir*:ti OR restrict*:ab OR restrict:ti OR consent*:ab OR consent*:ti OR
difficult*:ab OR difficult*:ti OR limitation*:ab OR limitation*:ti OR confidential*:ab
OR confidential*:ti OR privacy:ab OR privacy:ti OR distance*:ab OR distance*:ti OR
travel*:ab OR travel*:ti OR 'time factor'/exp OR time:ab OR time:ti OR delay*:ab
OR delay*:ti OR wait*:ab OR wait*:ti
AND
experienc*:ab OR experience*:ti OR perception*:ab OR perception*:ti OR
perceiv*:ab OR perceiv*:ti OR implication*:ab OR implication*:ti OR impact*:ab OR
impact*:ti OR perspective*:ab OR perspective*:ti OR influen*:ab OR influen*:ti OR
knowledge:ab OR knowledge:ti OR consequence*:ab OR consequence*:ti
AND
[humans]/lim

CANCER

Systematic Reviews and Primary Literature

Search Strategy: Cancer
Date: 2007–Present
Countries: United States and International
Population: Human
Document Types: Primary Literature, Editorials, Systematic Reviews, Meta-Analysis
Databases Searched: Medline, Embase, Cochrane, and PubMed

Search No.	Search Syntax
Medline (Ovid)	
1	Abortion, Induced/ or (induced adj abortion).ti,ab,kw.
2	abortion.ti,ab,kw.
3	(reproductive adj factors).ti,ab,kw.
4	(reproductive adj events).ti,ab,kw.
5	or/1–4
6	Neoplasms/ep [Epidemiology]
7	Neoplasms/
8	cancer.ti,ab,kw.

9	or/6–8
10	5 and 9
11	Animals/ or (animal or animals or mice or mouse or rat or rats).kw.
12	10 not 11
13	12
14	limit 13 to yr="2007–Current"
15	limit 14 to (meta analysis or "review" or systematic reviews)
16	limit 14 to (comment or editorial or letter)
17	14 not (15 or 16)

Embase (Ovid)

1	induced abortion/
2	(induced adj abortion).ti,ab,kw.
3	abortion.ti,ab,kw.
4	(reproductive adj factors).ti,ab,kw.
5	(reproductive adj events).ti,ab,kw.
6	or/1–4
7	malignant neoplasm/ep [Epidemiology]
8	malignant neoplasm/
9	cancer.ti,ab,kw.
10	or/7–9
11	6 and 10
12	Animals/ or (animal or animals or mice or mouse or rat or rats).kw.
13	11 not 12
14	13
15	limit 14 to yr="2007–Current"
16	limit 15 to (meta analysis or "systematic review")
17	limit 15 to (editorial or erratum or letter or note)
18	15 not (16 or 17)

Cochrane Database of Systematic Reviews (Ovid)

1	abortion.ti,ab,kw.
2	(reproductive adj events).ti,ab,kw.
3	(reproductive adj factors).ti,ab,kw.
4	cancer.ti,ab,kw.
5	1 and 4

PubMed:
("Abortion, Induced"[Mesh] OR abortion[Title/Abstract] OR "reproductive events"[Title/Abstract] OR "reproductive factors"[Title/Abstract] OR abortion[tw] OR "reproductive events"[tw] OR "reproductive factors"[tw]) AND ("Neoplasms"[Mesh] OR "Neoplasms/epidemiology"[Mesh] OR cancer[Title/Abstract] OR cancer[tw])
Date: 2007–Present
Limit: Humans

TRAINING

Systematic Reviews and Primary Literature

Database Searched and Time Period Covered:
PubMed: 1/1/2000–2/20/2017

Language:
English

Search Strategy:
"Abortion, Induced"[Mesh] OR abortion*[tiab] OR abortion*[ot]
AND
training OR trained OR competen* OR requirement* OR "Patient Safety"[Mesh] OR
"Professional Competence"[Mesh] OR safe[tiab] OR safety[tiab] OR unsafe
AND
AL[Affiliation] OR AK[Affiliation] OR AZ[Affiliation] OR AR[Affiliation] OR
CA[Affiliation] OR CO[Affiliation] OR CT[Affiliation] OR DE[Affiliation] OR
FL[Affiliation] OR GA[Affiliation] OR HI[Affiliation] OR ID[Affiliation] OR
IL[Affiliation] OR IN[Affiliation] OR IA[Affiliation] OR KS[Affiliation] OR
KY[Affiliation] OR LA[Affiliation] OR ME[Affiliation] OR MD[Affiliation] OR
MA[Affiliation] OR MI[Affiliation] OR MN[Affiliation] OR MS[Affiliation] OR
MO[Affiliation] OR MT[Affiliation] OR NE[Affiliation] OR NV[Affiliation] OR
NH[Affiliation] OR NJ[Affiliation] OR NM[Affiliation] OR NY[Affiliation] OR
NC[Affiliation] OR ND[Affiliation] OR OH[Affiliation] OR OK[Affiliation] OR
OR[Affiliation] OR PA[Affiliation] OR RI[Affiliation] OR SC[Affiliation] OR
SD[Affiliation] OR TN[Affiliation] OR TX[Affiliation] OR UT[Affiliation] OR
VT[Affiliation] OR VA[Affiliation] OR WA[Affiliation] OR WV[Affiliation] OR
WI[Affiliation] OR WY[Affiliation] OR USA[AFFILIATION] OR (Alabama[Affiliation]
OR Alaska[Affiliation] OR Arizona[Affiliation] OR Arkansas[Affiliation] OR
California[Affiliation] OR Colorado[Affiliation] OR Connecticut[Affiliation]
OR Delaware[Affiliation] OR Florida[Affiliation] OR Georgia[Affiliation]
OR Hawaii[Affiliation] OR Idaho[Affiliation] OR Illinois[Affiliation]
OR Indiana[Affiliation] OR Iowa[Affiliation] OR Kansas[Affiliation] OR
Kentucky[Affiliation] OR Louisiana[Affiliation] OR Maine[Affiliation] OR
Maryland[Affiliation] OR Massachusetts[Affiliation] OR Michigan[Affiliation] OR
Minnesota[Affiliation] OR Mississippi[Affiliation] OR Missouri[Affiliation] OR
Montana[Affiliation] OR Nebraska[Affiliation] OR Nevada[Affiliation] OR New
Hampshire[Affiliation] OR New Jersey[Affiliation] OR New Mexico[Affiliation] OR
New York[Affiliation] OR North Carolina[Affiliation] OR North Dakota[Affiliation]
OR Ohio[Affiliation] OR Oklahoma[Affiliation] OR Oregon[Affiliation] OR
Pennsylvania[Affiliation] OR Rhode Island[Affiliation] OR South Carolina[Affiliation]
OR South Dakota[Affiliation] OR Tennessee[Affiliation] OR Texas[Affiliation]
OR Utah[Affiliation] OR Vermont[Affiliation] OR Virginia[Affiliation] OR
Washington[Affiliation] OR West Virginia[Affiliation] OR Wisconsin[Affiliation] OR
Wyoming[Affiliation] OR united states[Affiliation])

Database Searched and Time Period Covered:
CINAHL: 1/1/2000–1/30/2017

Language:
English

Search Strategy:
MH "Abortion, Induced+") OR abortion*
AND
TI (training OR trained OR competen* OR requirement*) OR AB (training
OR trained OR competen* OR requirement*) OR MW (training OR trained OR
competen* OR requirement*)

Database Searched and Time Period Covered:
Cochrane: 1/1/2000–1/30/2017

Language:
English

Search Strategy:
MeSH descriptor: [Abortion, Induced] explode all trees OR abortion:ti,ab,kw (Word variations have been searched)
AND
training or trained or competen* or requirement*:ti,ab,kw (Word variations have been searched)